Copycat Recipes

Copycat Recipes- 2 Cookbooks In 1- A COMPLETE and EASY Step-By-Step Guide To Cook The Most Tasty And Famous Fast Food And Italian Recipes At Home.

MORE THEN 200 DISHES ARE WAITING FOR YOU!

Stacy Earls

© Copyright 2020 by Stacy Earls. All right reserved.

The work contained herein has been produced with the intent to provide relevant knowledge and information on the topic on the topic described in the title for entertainment purposes only. While the author has gone to every extent to furnish up to date and true information, no claims can be made as to its accuracy or validity as the author has made no claims to be an expert on this topic. Notwithstanding, the reader is asked to do their own research and consult any subject matter experts they deem necessary to ensure the quality and accuracy of the material presented herein.

This statement is legally binding as deemed by the Committee of Publishers Association and the American Bar Association for the territory of the United States. Other jurisdictions may apply their own legal statutes. Any reproduction, transmission or copying of this material contained in this work without the express written consent of the copyright holder shall be deemed as a copyright violation as per the current legislation in force on the date of publishing and subsequent time thereafter. All additional works derived from this material may be claimed by the holder of this copyright.

The data, depictions, events, descriptions and all other information forthwith are considered to be true, fair and accurate unless the work is expressly described as a work of fiction. Regardless of the nature of this work, the Publisher is exempt from any responsibility of actions taken by the reader in conjunction with this work. The Publisher acknowledges that the reader acts of their own accord and releases the author and Publisher of any responsibility for the observance of tips, advice, counsel, strategies and techniques that may be offered in this volume.

Table of Contents

INTRODUCTION	**15**
CHAPTER 1: MCDONALD'S™ SPECIALTIES	**19**
BREAKFAST	19
BREAKFAST BURRITO	19
EGG WHITE DELIGHT	21
LUNCH	23
CHEESEBURGER	23
CHICKEN MCNUGGETS	25
MCRIB SANDWICH	27
FILLET-O-FISH	29
DINNER	31
QUARTER-POUNDER WITH CHEESE	31
BEVERAGE OPTIONS	33
DELICIOUS SHAMROCK SHAKE	33
MCCAFE CARAMEL CAPPUCCINO	34
MCCAFE PEPPERMINT MOCHA	35
5-MINUTE PEPPERMINT MOCHA SYRUP	36
CHAPTER 2: BURGER KING™ SPECIALTIES	**37**
BREAKFAST	37
BK™ PANCAKE PLATTER	37
CINI MINIS	39
"EGG-NORMOUS" BURRITO	41
FRENCH TOAST STICKS	43
LUNCH	45
BK™ WHOPPER	45
CHICKEN FRIES	47
GRILLED CHICKEN SANDWICH	48
DINNER	50
CHICKEN GARDEN SALAD	50
RODEO KING	51

DESSERT	**54**
DUTCH APPLE PIE	54
OREO COOKIE CHEESECAKE	56

CHAPTER 3: CHEESECAKE FACTORY™ SPECIALTIES — **58**

BRUNCH	**58**
COBB SALAD DELIGHT	58
CRISPY CRAB CAKES	60
LUNCH OR DINNER	**62**
CUBAN SANDWICH SPECIALTY	62
FISH & CHIPS	63
FISH TACOS	65
GOAT CHEESE & BEET SALAD	67
MERLOT FILET MIGNON	69
PASTA DA VINCI	70
SOUTHERN-FRIED CATFISH	72
THE EVERYTHING PIZZA	73
WHITE CHICKEN CHILI	75
DESSERT	**77**
CARAMEL PECAN TURTLE CHEESECAKE	77
PUMPKIN CHEESECAKE	78

CHAPTER 4: TACO BELL™ SPECIALTIES — **80**

BREAKFAST	**80**
AM CRUNCHWRAP	80
CINNABON DELIGHTS	82
DRESSED EGG TACO	83
LUNCH	**85**
DELICIOUS TACOS	85
DINNER	**87**
CHALUPA SUPREME	87
GRILLED STEAK SOFT TACOS	89
XXL GRILLED STUFFED BURRITO	91
DESSERTS	**93**
TB BAJA BLAST FREEZE	93
TACO BELL CRISPITOS	94

CHAPTER 5: OLIVE GARDEN™ SPECIALTIES — **95**

BRUNCH	**95**
EGGPLANT PARMIGIANA	95
SHRIMP & CHICKEN CARBONARA	97
LUNCH	**99**
CHICKEN & GNOCCHI SOUP	99
MINESTRONE SOUP	101
DINNER	**103**
CHICKEN MARGHERITA	103
SHRIMP FETTUCCINE ALFREDO	105
DESSERT	**107**
RASPBERRY LEMONADE CONCENTRATE	107
TIRAMISU	109

CHAPTER 6: CHICK-FIL-A™ SPECIALTIES — **111**

BREAKFAST	**111**
CHICKEN BISCUIT	111
CHICKEN EGG & CHEESE BISCUIT	114
LUNCH	**117**
CHICK-FIL-A™ SANDWICH	117
MARKET SALAD	119
SWEET CARROT SALAD	121
DINNER	**122**
CHICK NUGGETS	122
HONEY MUSTARD GRILLED CHICKEN	124
DESSERT	**124**
BEST LEMONADE EVER	125
COOKIES & CREAM MILKSHAKE	126
PEPPERMINT MILKSHAKE	127

CHAPTER 7: DAIRY QUEEN™ SPECIALTIES — **128**

BRUNCH	**128**
CARAMEL MOOLATTE	128
TURKEY BLT	130

LUNCH	**132**
DQ FRIES	132
SLOW-COOKED CHILI CHEESE DOG	134
DINNER	**136**
FLAME-THROWER GRILL-BURGER	136
DESSERTS	**138**
DQ™ BANANA SPLIT	138
DQ™ ROUND CAKE	139
OREO COOKIE BLIZZARD	140
S'MORES BLIZZARD TREAT	141
VEGAN DQ CUPCAKES	142

CHAPTER 8: KFC™ SPECIALTIES   143

BRUNCH	**143**
GEORGIA GOLD FRIED CHICKEN	143
KFC™ BISCUITS	145
LUNCH	**146**
CREAMY COLESLAW	146
SLOW-COOKED MAC & CHEESE	147
DINNER	**148**
BBQ RODS	148
CHILI-LIME FRIED CHICKEN	150
KFC™ ORIGINAL-STYLE CHICKEN	152
SAUCES	**154**
KFC™ BUTTERMILK RANCH SAUCE	154
KFC™ SWEET N' TANGY BBQ SAUCE	156
DESSERT	**158**
CHOCOLATE CHIP CAKE	158

CHAPTER 9: BOJANGLES™ SPECIALTIES   160

BRUNCH	**160**
BO-BERRY BISCUIT	160
CHEDDAR BO BISCUIT	162
GRAVY BISCUIT	164
PLAIN BISCUIT SPECIALTY	165
STUFFED POTATO PANCAKES	166

LUNCH	**168**
DIRTY RICE	168
JAMBALAYA BOWL - SLOW-COOKED	169
DINNER	**171**
"BOJANGLER" ON-THE-GO	171
HOMESTYLE TENDERS	173
DESSERT	**174**
LEGENDARY BO SWEET ICED TEA CONCENTRATE	174
SWEET POTATO PIE	176

CHAPTER 10: STARBUCKS™ — **177**

BREAKFAST	**177**
BERRY TRIO YOGURT	177
CHOCOLATE CHUNK MUFFINS	179
EGG SALAD SANDWICH	181
SAUSAGE - CHEDDAR & EGG BREAKFAST SANDWICH	182
STARBUCKS™ PUMPKIN BREAD	184
LUNCH OR DINNER	**186**
ROASTED TOMATO & MOZZARELLA PANINI	186
TURKEY & HAVARTI SANDWICH	187
DESSERT	**188**
BLUEBERRY SCONE	188
CRANBERRY BLISS BAR	190
CRANBERRY ORANGE SCONE	192
ICED LEMON POUND CAKE	194
BEVERAGES	**196**
CHAI LATTE	196
HOT CHOCOLATE	198
ICED COCONUT MOCHA MACCHIATO	199
S'MORES FRAPPUCCINO	200
SALTED CARAMEL MOCHA	201

CHAPTER 11: SUBWAY™ SPECIALTIES — **203**

BREAKFAST	**203**
BMT SANDWICH	203
SUBWAY™ BREAD RECIPE	205
SUBWAY ™ SWEET ONION CHICKEN TERIYAKI SANDWICHES	207

LUNCH	**208**
ORCHARD CHICKEN SALAD	208
DINNER	**209**
MEATBALL SUB	209
DESSERT	**211**
CHEWY PEANUT BUTTER COOKIES	211
WHITE CHOCOLATE RASPBERRY COOKIES	213

CHAPTER 12: WENDY'S™ SPECIALTIES — **214**

BRUNCH	**214**
ARTISAN BACON EGG SANDWICH	214
BACONATOR	216
GRILLED ASIAGO RANCH CHICKEN CLUB	218
POWER MEDITERRANEAN CHICKEN SALAD	220
LUNCH	**222**
CHEESY STUFFED BAKED POTATO	222
CHILI - SLOW-COOKED	224
DAVE'S SINGLE	226
SPICY CHICKEN NUGGETS	226
DINNER	**227**
APPLE PECAN CHICKEN SALAD	228
TACO SALAD	230
DESSERT	**231**
DOUBLE CHOCOLATE CHIP COOKIES	231
FROSTY TIME	233

CONCLUSION — **234**

INTRODUCTION COPYCAT ITALIAN RECIPES — 237

CHAPTER 1: OLIVE GARDEN SPECIALITIES — 239

BRUNCH OPTIONS — **239**
ANGRY ALFREDO WITH CHICKEN — 239
BAKED PARMESAN SHRIMP — 241
TORTELLINI AL FORNO — 243
DINNER OPTIONS — **244**
BAKED TILAPIA & SHRIMP — 244
MANICOTTI — 246
RAVIOLI DI PORTOBELLO — 247
STEAK GORGONZOLA-ALFREDO — 249
SIDES — **251**
LASAGNA DIP & PASTA CHIPS — 251
PARMESAN ROASTED ASPARAGUS — 253
DESSERT — **255**
APPLE CARMELINA — 255
BEVERAGES — **256**
BERRY SANGRIA — 256
WATERMELON MOSCATO SANGRIA — 257

CHAPTER 2: CARRABBA'S ITALIAN GRILL — 258

BRUNCH OPTIONS — **258**
CHICKEN BRYAN — 258
LENTIL & SAUSAGE SOUP — 260
SICILIAN CHICKEN SOUP — 261
DINNER OPTIONS — **262**
DELICIOUS MEATBALLS — 262
LASAGNA — 264
MUSSELS IN WHITE WINE SAUCE — 266
SAUCES — **268**
THE GRILL'S SEASONING — 268
ITALIAN BUTTER — 269

CHAPTER 3: BIAGGI'S RISTORANTE ITALIANO RESTAURANT   **270**

BRUNCH OPTIONS	**270**
FORMAGGI DI CAPRA	270
MUSHROOM CHICKEN ALFREDO	272
RAVIOLI ROMANO	273
TUSCAN COUNTRY SALAD	275
DINNER OPTIONS	**276**
GARMUGIA SOUP	276
PORK CHOPS MILANESE	277
SAUCE	**279**
ALFREDO SAUCE	279
SIDE DISH	**280**
BISCOTTI DI PRATO	280
DESSERT	**281**
BIAGGI'S RISTORANTE ITALIANO BAROLO ZABAIONE	281

CHAPTER 4: FAZOLI'S FAVORITES   **282**

BRUNCH OPTIONS	**282**
GRILLED CHICKEN PANINI	282
STUFFED SEAFOOD SHELLS	284
DINNER OPTIONS	**286**
BAKED BEEF & SPAGHETTI	286
BAKED GARLIC CHICKEN SPAGHETTI	288
SIDE DISH	**290**
DELICIOUS BREADSTICKS	290

CHAPTER 5: ORIGINAL SICILIAN PASTA CO.   **291**

BRUNCH OPTION	**291**
CALABRESE	291
DINNER OPTIONS	**292**
CALAMARI BOLOGNESE	292
PARTY TIME SICILIAN PASTA SHRIMP ALFREDO	293
SIDES	**294**
PARTY-TIME BRUSCHETTA SPREAD	294
STUFFED PORTOBELLOS	295

CHAPTER 6: PASTA HOUSE COMPANY — **297**

BRUNCH OPTIONS	**297**
FETTUCCINE ALFREDO	297
PASTA CON BROCCOLI	298
PENNE PRIMAVERA	299
DINNER OPTIONS	**300**
CHICKEN FLAMINGO	300
CHICKEN IGNATIO	302
SIDES	**303**
GARLIC CHEESE BREAD	303
PASTA HOUSE CO. SPECIAL SALAD	304

CHAPTER 7: ROMANO'S MACARONI GRILL — **305**

BRUNCH OPTION	**305**
PESTO CHICKEN FARFALLE	305
DINNER OPTIONS	**307**
MACARONI GRILL SEAFOOD LINGUINE	307
PASTA DI MARE	309
PENNE RUSTICA	311

CHAPTER 8: NYC RESTAURANT FAVORITES — **313**

BRUNCH OPTIONS	**313**
CARMINES ITALIAN SALAD	313
SICILIAN PEPPERONI PIZZA AT PRINCE STREET PIZZA	315
SPICY HONEY SOPPRESSATA PIZZA " THE BEE STING PIZZA" AT ROBERTA'S PIZZERIA	316
DINNER OPTIONS	**317**
CARMINE'S BAKED CLAMS	317
CARMINE'S CHICKEN PARMIGIANA	318
SPICY VODKA RIGATONI AT MARIO CARBONE'S	320

CHAPTER 9: THE OLD SPAGHETTI FACTORY — **322**

BRUNCH OPTIONS	**322**
CHICKEN TETRAZZINI	322
SPAGHETTI WITH BURNT BUTTER	324

DINNER OPTION	**325**
BEER CHILI	325
SAUCE FAVORITE	**326**
CREAMY PESTO SALAD DRESSING	326

CHAPTER 10: ZIO'S ITALIAN KITCHEN — 327

BRUNCH OPTIONS	**327**
CHICKEN PEPPERONI	327
TOMATO FLORENTINE SOUP	329
DINNER OPTION	**331**
CHICKEN POMODORO	331
SIDES	**332**
ARTICHOKE SPINACH DIP	332
BREAD DIPPING OIL	334
ITALIAN NACHOS	335
ZIO'S SPICE MIX	337

CHAPTER 11: VARIETY RESTAURANTS - COPYCAT RECIPES — 338

BRUNCH OPTIONS	**338**
GODFATHER'S ANTIPASTO SALAD/PARTY TRAY	338
GODFATHER'S DEEP DISH PIZZA	340
UNO'S CHICAGO GRILL SHRIMP SCAMPI PASTA	341
DINNER OPTIONS	**342**
TACO PIZZA BY PIZZA INN	342
SIDES	**343**
PAPA JOHN'S GARLIC KNOTS	343
THE SPAGHETTI WAREHOUSE MEAT SAUCE	344
SERVINGS: 6-8 | DIFFICULTY: SUPER-EASY | TIME: 2.5 HOURS	344
DESSERTS	**345**
CI CI'S CHERRY DESSERT PIZZA	345
CI CI'S CHOCOLATE DESSERT PIZZA	346
GODFATHER'S PIZZA: CINNAMON STREUSEL DESSERT PIZZA	347
BEVERAGE FAVORITE	**348**
THE SPAGHETTI WAREHOUSE SANGRIA	348

CONCLUSION — 349

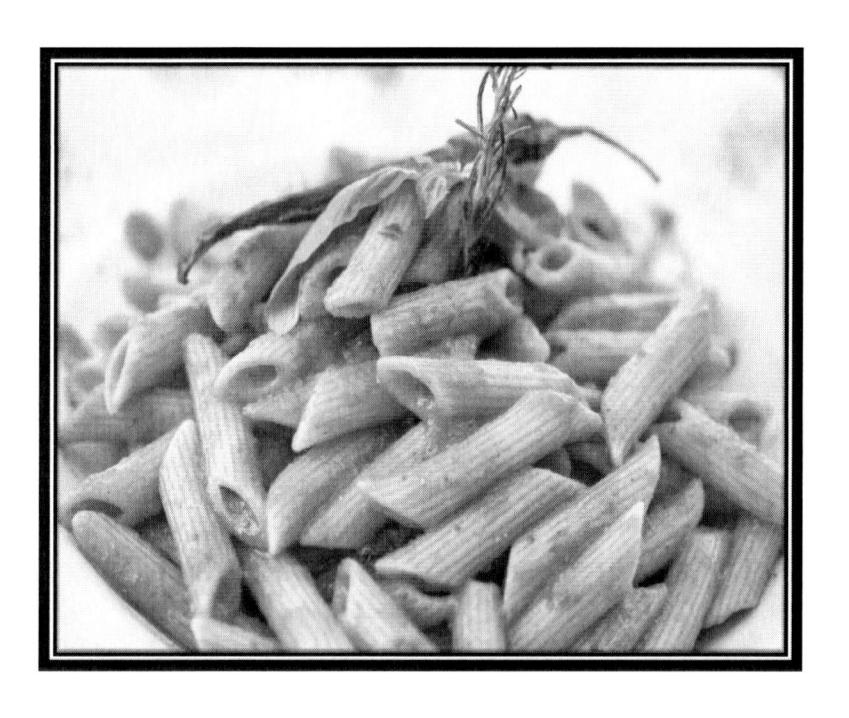

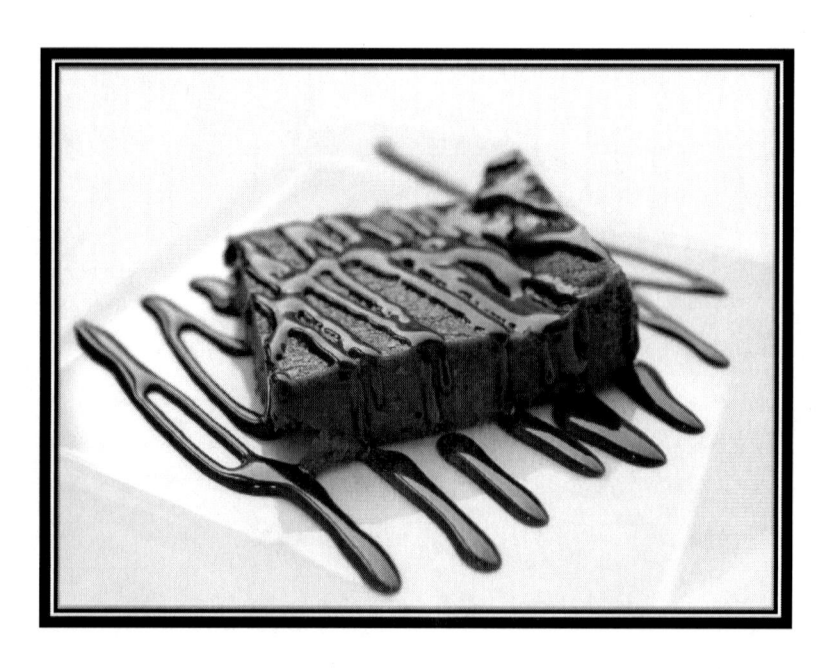

Introduction

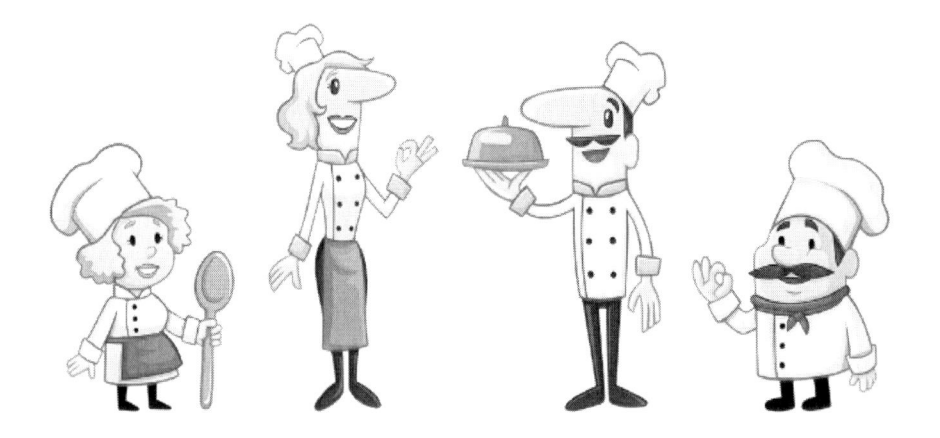

Congratulations on purchasing *Copycat Recipes,* and thank you for doing so. Not only will you be acquiring a batch of new recipes for your friends and family, but you will also be gaining many other benefits.

The following chapters will discuss a variety of delicious recipes copied from your favorite restaurants, including:

- McDonald's
- Burger King
- Cheesecake Factory
- Taco Bell™
- Olive Garden
- Chick-fil-A™

- Long John Silvers™
- KFC™
- Bojangles™
- Starbucks™ Drinks Galore
- Subway™
- Wendy's™

These are just a few of improvements you will achieve during your new dining experience.

- *Replicate Your Favorite Dishes From The Best Restaurants At Home, Saving Your Money.*
- *Save A Lot Of Time By Avoiding Unnecessary Lines At The Checkout.*
- *Eat Your Favorite Dishes In The Comfort Of Your Home.*
- *Improve Your Cooking Skills.*
- *Consume Healthier Ingredients.*
- *Elimination Of Ingredients That May Cause Food Allergies.*
- *Use More Natural Preparation Methods To Prepare Your Favorite Recipes.*
- *Maximize Portion Control.*
- *Benefits Your Health.*
- *Have Greater Control Of Your Diet.*

- *Improved Eating Habits Are Possible.*
- *Amaze Your Family And Friends With The Most Popular Restaurant Dishes.*

You will soon better understand the type of tools and accessories needed to prepare your copycat delights! You will want to be sure you correctly measure your products as you follow the set of guidelines provided.

Begin with a good set of scales with a conversion button. You need to know how to convert measurements into grams since not all recipes have them listed. The grams keep the system in complete harmony. Choose a set of scales with a tare function. When you set a bowl on the scale, the feature will allow you to reset the weight back to zero (0). Keep the germs off of the scale with the use of a removable plate. Be sure it will come off (before purchasing) to eliminate any bacterial buildup.

These are a few more vital tools you will need to compete with the pro's guidelines:

- **Wire cooling racks** are useful in cooling bread, muffins, and many other dishes.

- ***Sifter****:* Purchase a good sifter for under $10, and you will be ensured a more accurate measurement for your baking needs.

- **Cutting boards** are used during many phases of prep. Consider having different colored heavy-duty plastic boards for each type of food item to help prevent cross-contamination.

- **Measuring cups** are needed for liquid and dry ingredients.

- ***Measuring spoons*** are essential for a successful dish. If you do a lot of baking and cooking, consider a magnetic set, so the spoon is never lost, and they will also fit into spice jars.

- ***Whisks*** can be purchased in different sizes and are used in many recipes.

- ***Sheet Pans***: A baking tray can quickly become one of the most used items in the kitchen as you prepare your delicious copycat recipes. You can bake meat, roast veggies, toast nuts, and make trays of delicious sweets.

- ***Saucepans***: Boiling vegetables and pasta will require a pan that's easily maneuvered when filled. Start with a four-quart pan, whether you are cooking for one or four.

- ***Non-Stick Frying Pan***: A non-stick pan is vital if you want to deliver a delicious and eye-appealing egg meal as the big restaurants provide. You can also sauté veggies, sear meats, and prepare delicious sauces. Have two sizes on hand, so you can make different steps of the recipes (save time too).

You will also want to have a dampened tea towel, plastic wrap, and a package of parchment baking paper. This is a fairly accurate list of the accessories you will need to begin your new cooking adventure.

Let's Get Started!

Chapter 1: McDonald's™ Specialties

Breakfast

Breakfast Burrito

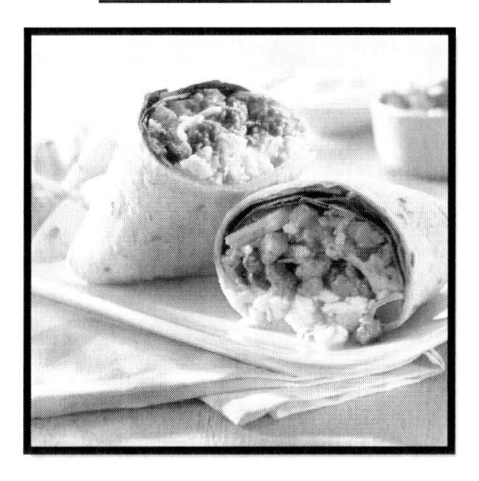

Servings: 10 | **Difficulty**: Easy | **Time**: 35 min

Nutrition per Serving:

- Calories: 269
- Protein: 15 grams
- Fat Content: 21 grams
- Sat. Fats: 8 grams
- Carbohydrates: 3 grams
- Sugars: 1 gram
- Fiber: 0 grams

Ingredients Needed:

- ☐ Mild pork sausage (1 lb.)
- ☐ Yellow onion (.5 cup)
- ☐ Fresh tomatoes (.25 cup)
- ☐ Green - canned chiles (1 tbsp.)
- ☐ Tortillas (10)
- ☐ Eggs (9)
- ☐ American sliced cheese (6 oz.)
- ☐ Salsa (.5 cup.)

Preparation Guidelines:

1. Crumble and fry the sausage, stirring to separate into small little pieces. Transfer the pan to a cool burner and drain the excess grease.
2. Toss the drained sausage into a skillet. Mince and add green chilies, onion, and tomatoes. Warm the pan and sauté them using the medium temperature setting until the veggies and sausage are thoroughly heated. Stir often.
3. Measure and whisk in the eggs. Add them to the pan with the sausage mixture. When cooked, remove the pan from heat.
4. Place two tablespoons of the sausage and egg mixture onto a tortilla, tear each slice of American cheese into two even portions, then add the cheese, and roll the tortilla.
5. If you make these all ahead of time, you can wrap in plastic and pop into the fridge or freezer. Heat the burritos in the microwave for a minute or two.
6. Serve with your favorite taco or Picante sauce, sour cream, or avocado.

Egg White Delight

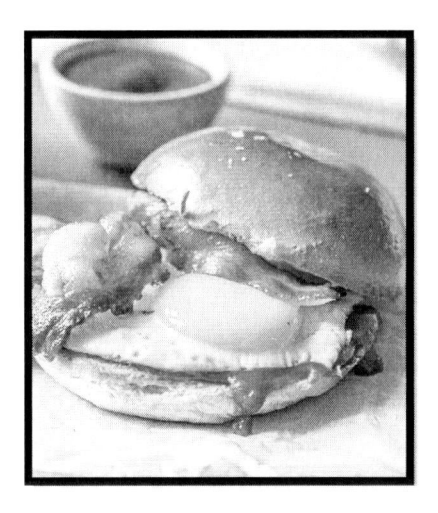

Servings: 2 | **Difficulty**: Easy | **Time**: 10 min

Nutrition per Serving:

- Calories: 195
- Protein: 17 grams
- Fat Content: 3 grams
- Sat. Fats: 1 gram
- Carbohydrates: 23 grams
- Sugars: 5 grams
- Fiber: 3 grams

Ingredients Needed:

- ☐ English muffins (2 wheat)
- ☐ Canadian bacon (2 slices)
- ☐ Egg whites (4)
- ☐ Black pepper & salt (as desired)
- ☐ Cheddar/low-fat cheese (2 slices)

Preparation Guidelines:

1. Toast the muffins in a toaster.
2. Warm a skillet to cook the bacon until it's slightly browned and remove it from the skillet.
3. Separate the yolks of the eggs for another recipe. Whisk the egg whites, pepper, and salt.
4. Spritz the pan using a portion of cooking oil spray and add the eggs. Adjust the temperature setting to low to cook the egg whites.
5. When the egg whites have cooked, assemble the sandwiches, and serve.

Lunch

Cheeseburger

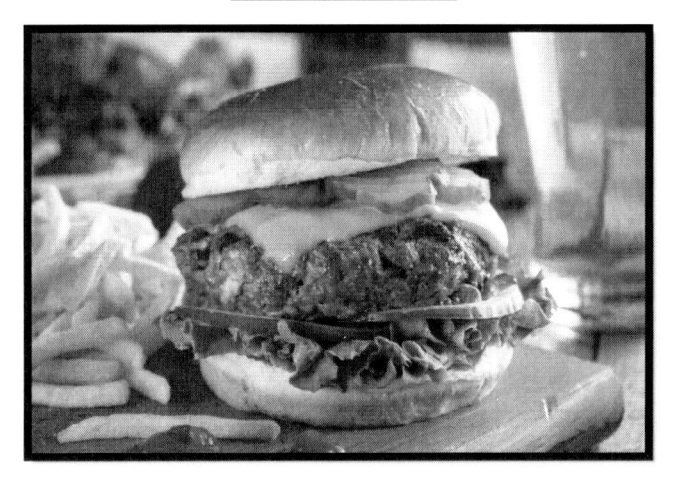

Servings: 4 | **Difficulty**: Easy | **Time**: 30 min

Nutrition per Serving:

- Calories: 403
- Fat: 17 grams
- Sat. Fats: 6 grams
- Protein: 18 grams
- Fiber: 1 gram
- Sugars: 6 grams

Ingredients Needed:

- ☐ Steak sauce (.25 cup)
- ☐ Seasoned coating mix - divided (2 tbsp. + 1/3 cup)
- ☐ Ground beef (1 lb.)
- ☐ Burger buns (4 - split)
- ☐ Lettuce leaves (4)

Preparation Guidelines:

1. Combine the two tablespoons of the coating mix with steak sauce and mix it with the beef and shape it into four 3.5-inch patties. Dip each of the patties in the rest of the coating mixture.
2. Arrange the prepared patties onto an ungreased baking tray.
3. Set the oven temperature at 350 °Fahrenheit until an internal thermometer reads 160 °Fahrenheit (20 min.), flipping them once.
4. Serve on toasted or untoasted buns with a portion of lettuce.

Chicken McNuggets

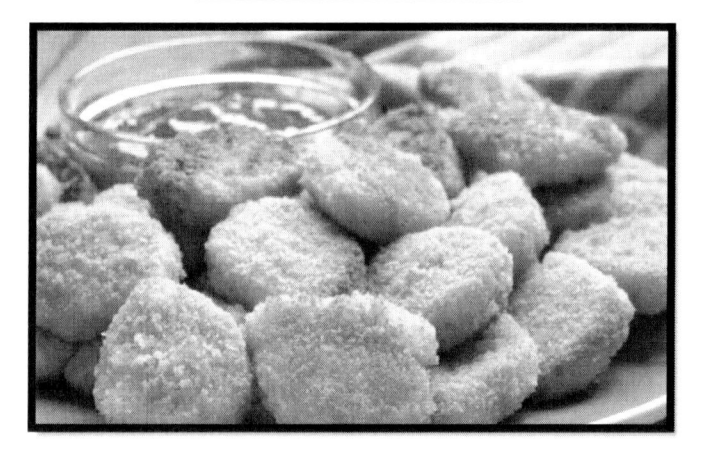

Servings: 8 | **Difficulty**: Easy | **Time**: 30 min

Nutrition per Serving: 6 nuggets - without sauce:

- Calories: 191
- Protein: 20 grams
- Fat: 9 grams
- Sat. Fats: 5 grams
- Carbohydrates: 5 grams
- Sugars: 0 grams
- Fiber: 0 grams

Ingredients Needed:

- ☐ Melted butter (.25 cup)
- ☐ Breadcrumbs (1 cup)
- ☐ Parmesan cheese (.5 cup - grated)
- ☐ Kosher salt (.5 tsp.)
- ☐ Chicken breast (1-inch cubes / 1.5 lb.)
- ☐ Optional: Marinara sauce (as desired)
- ☐ Also Needed: Two 15x10x1-inch baking pan

Preparation Guidelines:

1. Warm the oven to reach 375 °Fahrenheit.
2. Melt and pour the butter in a shallow mixing container.
3. Toss the breadcrumbs, cheese, and salt in another shallow container.
4. Dip the chicken in butter, and roll it in the crumbs.
5. Arrange each piece on the pans (not touching).
6. Set a timer to bake for 15-18 minutes, turning once. (It should no longer be pink inside.).
7. Serve with marinara sauce if desired.
8. Freeze leftovers if desired. Let the nuggets cool thoroughly and freeze in heavy-duty bags or other freezer containers. Partially thaw in the fridge overnight. Place on a baking sheet and set the oven at 375 °Fahrenheit oven 7-12 minutes or until hot as desired.

McRib Sandwich

Servings: 8 | **Difficulty**: Easy | **Time**: 6.5 hours

Nutrition per Serving:
- Calories: 405
- Protein: 26 grams
- Fat: 13 grams
- Sat. Fats: 4 grams
- Carbohydrates: 45 grams
- Sugars: 13 grams
- Fiber: 2 grams

Ingredients Needed:
- ☐ Large onion (1)
- ☐ Country-style boneless pork ribs (2 lb.)
- ☐ Ketchup (.5 cup)
- ☐ Plum sauce (.25 cup)
- ☐ Chili sauce (.25 cup)
- ☐ Garlic powder (1 tsp.)
- ☐ Brown sugar (2 tbsp.)
- ☐ Celery seed (1 tsp.)
- ☐ Optional: Liquid smoke (1 tsp.)
- ☐ Ground allspice (.5 tsp.)
- ☐ Split kaiser rolls (8)
- ☐ Also Needed: 3-qt. slow cooker

Preparation Guidelines:

1. Chop and toss the onion into the cooker. Top with ribs. Combine the plum sauce, ketchup, brown sugar, chili sauce, garlic powder, celery seed, allspice, and liquid smoke -if desired - and pour it over ribs.
2. Securely close the lid and set the timer for six to seven hours using the low-temperature setting. It should be tender.
3. Shred the meat by hand or with two forks. Serve the delicious meat on rolls and enjoy them in your "own" kitchen.

Fillet-O-Fish

Servings: 4 | **Difficulty**: Easy | **Time**: 30 min

Nutrition per Serving:

- Calories: 337
- Protein: 41 grams
- Fat: 7 grams
- Sat. Fats: 1 gram
- Carbohydrates: 28 grams
- Sugars: 5 grams
- Fiber: 4 grams

Ingredients Needed:

- ☐ Dry breadcrumbs (.5 cup)
- ☐ Garlic powder (.5 tsp.)
- ☐ Lemon pepper seasoning (.25 tsp.)
- ☐ Paprika (.5 tsp.)
- ☐ Cayenne pepper (.5 tsp.)
- ☐ Cod/halibut fillets (4@ 6 oz. each)
- ☐ Lettuce (1 cup)
- ☐ Carrots (.25 cup)
- ☐ Optional: Onion (1 tbsp.)

The Sauce:
- ☐ Plain yogurt (.25 cup)
- ☐ Lemon juice (1 tbsp.)
- ☐ Dill weed (.5 tsp.)
- ☐ Grated lemon zest (.25 tsp.)
- ☐ Garlic powder (.25 tsp.)
- ☐ Prepared horseradish (.25 tsp.)

Preparation Guidelines:

1. Shred the carrots and lettuce. Grate the onion.
2. Combine the breadcrumbs, garlic powder, paprika, lemon seasoning, and cayenne in a shallow dish (up to the line). Coat the fillets with the breadcrumb mixture.
3. Lightly spritz the grilling rack using cooking oil. Grill the fish with the lid on, using the medium temperature setting or broil in the oven for four to five minutes per side. Test for doneness by flaking it using a fork; if it flakes easily, it is done.
4. Grill the buns with the cut side down, using the medium temperature setting for 30-60 seconds until they are lightly toasted as you like them.
5. Prepare the lettuce, carrots, and onion as desired. In a separate container, combine the sauce fixings, and spread it over the bun bottoms. Top it with the fish and veggie mixture, and replace bun tops.

Dinner

Quarter-Pounder With Cheese

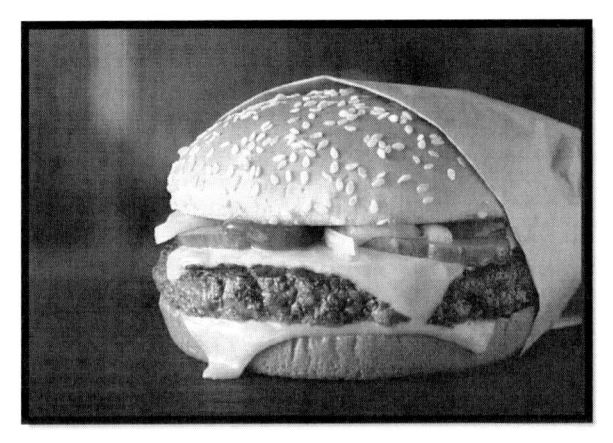

Servings: 4 | **Difficulty**: Easy | **Time**: 25 min

Nutrition per Serving:

- Calories: 429
- Carbohydrates: 32 grams
- Protein: 28 grams
- Fat: 20 grams
- Sat. Fats: 6 grams
- Sugars: 3 grams
- Fiber: 1 gram

Ingredients Needed:
- ☐ Seasoned breadcrumbs (.5 cup)
- ☐ Lightly whisked egg (1 large)
- ☐ Pepper and salt (.5 tsp. each)
- ☐ Ground beef (1 lb.)
- ☐ Olive oil (1 tbsp.)
- ☐ Sesame seed burger buns - split (4)
- ☐ Toppings of preference

Preparation Guidelines:

1. Combine the egg, breadcrumbs, salt, and pepper. Add and shape the beef mixture into four ½-inch thick patties. Make an indention with your thumb in the center of each one and brush them using a portion of oil.
2. Grill the burgers with the top on, using the medium temperature setting for four to five minutes per side (internal temp of 160 °Fahrenheit).
3. Arrange the burger on the buns using toppings to your liking.

Beverage Options

Delicious Shamrock Shake

Servings: 2 | **Difficulty**: Easy | **Time**: 5 min

Nutrition per Serving: 2/3 cup portion:

- Calories: 363
- Protein: 3 grams
- Fat: 12 grams
- Sat. Fats: 7 grams
- Carbohydrates: 49 grams
- Sugars: 47 grams
- Fiber: 1 gram

Ingredients Needed:

- ☐ Creme de Menthe/2% milk (3 tbsp + 1 dash of peppermint extract)
- ☐ Vanilla ice cream (1.25-1.5 cups)
- ☐ Thin Mint - Girl Scout cookies (7)
- ☐ Optional: Green food coloring

Preparation Guidelines:

1. Toss each of the fixings into a blender.
2. Place the lid and process until thoroughly mixed.
3. Enjoy immediately.

McCafe Caramel Cappuccino

Servings: 1 | **Difficulty**: Easy | **Time**: 8 min

Nutrition per Serving:

- Calories: 212
- Protein: 5 grams
- Fat Content: 8 grams
- Sat. Fats: 4 grams
- Carbohydrates: 29 grams
- Sugars: 26 grams

Ingredients Needed:

- ☐ Strong coffee (6 oz.) or Espresso (2 shots)
- ☐ Milk - low-fat (.5 cup)
- ☐ Caramel ice cream topping - divided (2 tbsp.)
- ☐ To Garnish: Whipped cream (2 tbsp.)

Preparation Guidelines:

1. Prepare the coffee in a hot mug.
2. Add one tablespoon of syrup and the warmed milk to the cup.
3. Garnish it with the whipped cream and a drizzle of the syrup.

McCafe Peppermint Mocha

Servings: 1 | **Difficulty**: Easy | **Time**: 10 min

Nutrition per Serving:

- Calories: 244
- Protein: 8 grams
- Fat Content: 10 grams
- Sat. Fats: 5 grams
- Carbohydrates: 29 grams
- Sugars: 25 grams

Ingredients Needed:

- ☐ Peppermint mocha syrup - see below (1-2 tbsp.)
- ☐ Coffee or espresso shot (1 cup)
- ☐ Milk - steamed (1 cup)
- ☐ Whipped cream (2 tbsp.)
- ☐ Chocolate syrup (1 tsp.)

Preparation Guidelines:

1. Measure and add the peppermint syrup in a coffee mug with the coffee.
2. Stir in heated milk.
3. Top with whipped cream and syrup to your liking.

5-Minute Peppermint Mocha Syrup

Servings: 16 tablespoons | **Difficulty**: Easy | **Time**: 5 min

Ingredients Needed:

- ☐ Water (.5 cup)
- ☐ Sugar (1 cup)
- ☐ Cocoa powder (2 tbsp.)
- ☐ Peppermint extract (.25 tsp.)

Preparation Guidelines:

1. Whisk the cocoa, sugar, and water in a saucepan using the medium temperature setting.
2. Boil it for one minute and remove it from the burner to add the peppermint.
3. Once the syrup is cooled, store it in the fridge. Enjoy the thickened syrup now and save the rest of it for another time.

Chapter 2: Burger King™ Specialties

Breakfast

BK™ Pancake Platter

Servings: 2.5 dozen | **Difficulty**: Easy | **Time**: 15-20 min

Nutrition per Serving - 3 pancakes:

- Calories: 270
- Protein: 11 grams
- Fat: 3 grams
- Sat. Fats: 1 gram
- Carbohydrates: 48 grams
- Sugars: 11 grams
- Fiber: 1 gram

Ingredients Needed:

- ☐ Baking powder (1.5 tsp.)
- ☐ A-P flour (4 cups)
- ☐ Baking soda (2 tsp.)
- ☐ Sugar (.25 cup)
- ☐ Salt (2 tsp.)
- ☐ Unchilled eggs (4 large)
- ☐ Buttermilk (4 cups)

Preparation Guidelines:

1. Whisk the baking soda, flour, salt, baking powder, and sugar.
2. Use another container to beat the buttermilk and room temperature eggs. Stir the mixture into dry fixings just until moistened.
3. Pour the batter (¼ cup each) onto a lightly greased hot griddle. Flip each of the cakes once bubbles appear.
4. Flip and continue cooking until they're done.
5. Garnish with your favorite toppings and serve.

Cini Minis

Servings: 2 dozen | **Difficulty**: Medium | **Time**: 40 min

Nutrition per Serving:

- Calories: 176
- Protein: 3 grams
- Fat: 7 grams
- Sat. Fats: 4 grams
- Carbohydrates: 26 grams
- Fiber: 1 gram
- Sugars: 14 grams

Ingredients Needed:

- ☐ Whole milk (.66 cup)
- ☐ Maple syrup (.33 cup)
- ☐ Unchilled butter (.33 cup)
- ☐ Large egg (1)
- ☐ Bread flour (3 cups.)
- ☐ Salt (.75 tsp.)
- ☐ Active dry yeast (¼ oz. pkg.)

The Topping:
- ☐ Brown sugar (.5 cup - tightly packed)
- ☐ Bread flour (2 tbsp.)
- ☐ Cinnamon (4 tsp.)
- ☐ Cold butter (6 tbsp.)

The Icing:
- ☐ Whole milk (1-2 tsp.)
- ☐ Confectioner's sugar (1 cup)
- ☐ Maple syrup (3 tbsp.)
- ☐ Butter (3 tbsp.)
- ☐ Also Needed: Bread Machine & Greased 13x9-inch baking pan.

Preparation Guidelines:

1. Measure and add the first seven fixings into the bread machine. Choose the dough setting, checking it after about five minutes of mixing. Mix in flour or water as needed.
2. When the time has elapsed, flip the dough onto a cutting board/countertop dusted with flour.
3. Roll the dough into two 12 by 7-inch rectangles. Sift/whisk the flour, cinnamon, and brown sugar. Sprinkle half over each rectangle and roll them up, pinching to seal.
4. Slice the rolls into twelve slices and arrange them into the baking pan. Place a lid on the pan and put it in a warm space to rise until it is about doubled in size (20 min.).
5. Warm the oven and bake it at 375° Fahrenheit until golden brown (20-25 min.). Wait for about five minutes after you place it onto a cooling rack.
6. Mix the syrup, confectioners' sugar, milk, and butter until it's spreadable for the warm rolls.

"Egg-normous" Burrito

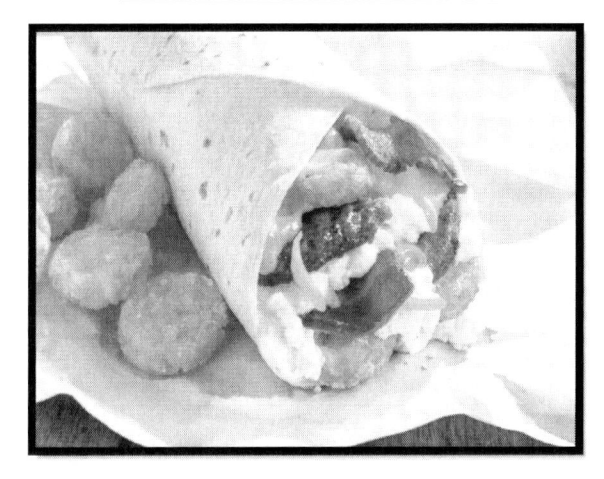

Servings: 10 | **Difficulty**: Easy | **Time**: 4.5 hours

Nutrition per Serving:

- Calories: 683
- Protein: 35 grams
- Fat: 38 grams
- Sat. Fats: 15 grams
- Carbohydrates: 41 grams
- Sugars: 3 grams
- Fiber: 7 grams

Ingredients Needed:

- [ ] Pork sausage (1 lb. bulk)
- [ ] Bacon strips (.5 lb.)
- [ ] Large eggs (18)
- [ ] Frozen hash brown shredded potatoes (2 cups)
- [ ] Onion (1 large - chopped)
- [ ] Condensed - cheddar cheese soup (1 can - undiluted - 10.75 oz.)
- [ ] Green chiles (4 oz, can - chopped)
- [ ] Pepper (.5 tsp.)
- [ ] Garlic powder (1 tsp.)

- ☐ Shredded cheddar cheese (2 cups)
- ☐ Warmed flour tortillas (10 - 10-inch)

Optional Toppings:
- ☐ Salsa
- ☐ Jalapeno peppers
- ☐ Hot pepper sauce
- ☐ Also Needed: Four or five-quart slow cooker

Preparation Guidelines:

1. Mix the sausage, bacon, hash browns, eggs, onions, soup, chiles, pepper, and garlic powder (up to the line). Prepare as below.
2. Thaw and shred the hash browns. Cook and drain the sausage and bacon on a layer of paper towels. Whisk and add the eggs with the bacon, sausage, potatoes, onion, and soup.
3. Dump about half of the egg mixture into the cooker coated with a cooking oil spray. Top the mix and reserve half of the cheese. Repeat the layers.
4. Cook, covered, using the low function for four to five hours or until the center is set.
5. Spoon about ¾ cup of egg mixture across the center of each tortilla.
6. Fold the bottom and sides of the tortilla over the filling and roll it up.
7. Add toppings of your choice.

French Toast Sticks

Servings: 1.5 dozen | **Difficulty**: Easy | **Time**: 40 min

Nutrition per Serving - 3 each serving:

- Calories: 183
- Carbohydrates: 24 grams
- Protein: 8 grams
- Fat: 6 grams
- Sat. Fats: 2 grams
- Fiber: 1 gram
- Sugars: 8 grams

Ingredients Needed:

- ☐ Texas toast slices (6 day-olds)
- ☐ Large eggs (4)
- ☐ 2% milk (1 cup)
- ☐ Cinnamon (.25-.5 tsp.)
- ☐ Sugar (2 tbsp.)
- ☐ Vanilla extract (1 tsp.)

Optional Ingredients:
- ☐ Crushed cornflakes (1 cup)
- ☐ Confectioner's sugar
- ☐ Maple syrup
- ☐ Also Needed: 15x10x1-inch baking pan

Preparation Guidelines:

1. Slice each piece of bread into thirds and arrange them in an ungreased pan.
2. Whisk the milk, sugar, eggs, vanilla, and cinnamon. Dump it over the bread and soak for about two minutes, flipping once. Coat the dough with cornflake crumbs.
3. Place in a greased baking pan. Freeze the sticks until firm (45 min.). Transfer to an airtight freezer container and store in the freezer.
4. When it's time to eat, add and bake them at 425 °Fahrenheit for eight minutes. Flip them over and cook f until golden brown (10-12 min.). Sprinkle them using the confectioners' sugar and serve with syrup.

Lunch

BK™Whopper

Servings: 4 | **Difficulty**: Easy | **Time**: 20 min

Nutrition per Serving:

- Calories: 526
- Protein: 24 grams
- Fat: 34 grams
- Sat. Fats: 10 grams
- Carbohydrates: 27 grams
- Sugars: 7 grams
- Fibers: 1 gram

Ingredients Needed:

- ☐ Ground chuck (1 lb.)
- ☐ Black pepper (.25 tsp.)
- ☐ Salt (.5 tsp.)
- ☐ Sesame burger buns (4)
- ☐ Pickle slices (12)
- ☐ Mayo (4 tbsp.)
- ☐ Ketchup (4 tbsp.)
- ☐ White onion (half of 1)

Preparation Guidelines:

1. Slice the onions and tomatoes.
2. Prepare the beef with pepper and salt, shaping it into patties.
3. Butter and toast the buns until browned using the med-high temperature setting.
4. Simmer the burger for 2-3 minutes per side, sprinkling with salt as desired.
5. Prepare the burger with the meat on the bottom. Continue to layer it using three to four slices of pickle, three to four rings of onion, and two to three slices of tomato. Squirt it with ketchup, and add lettuce and mayo. Add the top of the bun and serve.

Chicken Fries

Servings: 4 | **Difficulty**: Easy | **Time**: 35 min

Nutrition per Serving:
- Calories: 376
- Protein: 22.1 grams
- Fat: 17 grams
- Sat. Fats: 6 grams
- Carbohydrates: 27 grams
- Sugars: 1 gram
- Fiber: 2 grams

Ingredients Needed:
- ☐ Whisked eggs (2 large)
- ☐ Cayenne pepper (.5-.25 tsp.)
- ☐ Salt (.5 tsp.)
- ☐ Garlic powder (.5 tsp.)
- ☐ Ridged potato chips (2 cups)
- ☐ Grated parmesan cheese (.5 cup)
- ☐ Panko breadcrumbs (1 cup)
- ☐ Skinless-boneless chicken (2 breasts/6 oz. each @ ¼-inch strips)

Preparation Guidelines:
1. Warm the oven at 400° Fahrenheit.
2. Use a shallow mixing container to whisk the eggs, salt, garlic powder, and cayenne.
3. In another shallow bowl, crush and combine the breadcrumbs, chips, and cheese.
4. Dredge the pieces of chicken in the egg mixture and the potato chip mixture - patting to help the coating adhere.
5. Transfer them onto a greased wire rack in a foil-lined rimmed baking sheet.
6. Bake until golden brown (12-15 min.).

Grilled Chicken Sandwich

Servings: 4 | **Difficulty**: Easy | **Time**: 30 min

Nutrition per Serving:

- Calories: 490
- Carbohydrates: 32 grams
- Protein: 30 grams
- Fat: 27 grams
- Sat. Fats: 15 grams
- Sugars: 2 grams
- Fibers: 2 grams

Ingredients Needed:

- ☐ Chicken breast halves - boneless-no skin (4 @ 4 oz. each)
- ☐ Butter - divided (6 tbsp.)
- ☐ Garlic clove (1)
- ☐ Dill weed - divided (.75 tsp.)
- ☐ Softened cream cheese (.25 cup)
- ☐ French bread slices (8 @ .5-inch thick)
- ☐ Lemon juice (2 tsp.)
- ☐ Lettuce leaves (4)
- ☐ Tomato (8 slices)

Preparation Guidelines:

1. Flatten chicken to ¼-inch thickness.
2. Mince and sauté the garlic in a large skillet. Mix in ¼ teaspoon dill and three tablespoons butter and sauté them for one minute. Add chicken and cook using medium heat until the juices run clear when poked with a fork (3-4 min.) per side. Remove and keep warm.
3. Spread both sides of the bread using the rest of the butter. Grill the bread on both sides until browned to your liking.
4. Combine the lemon juice, cream cheese, and remaining dill (½ tsp.) and spread it on one side of grilled bread.
5. Arrange the lettuce, chicken, and tomato on four slices of bread. Top it off with the remaining slices of bread.

Dinner

Chicken Garden Salad

Servings: 8 | **Difficulty**: Very Easy | **Time**: 30 min

Nutrition per Serving:
- Calories: 380
- Protein: 15 grams
- Fat: 31 grams
- Sat. Fats: 8 grams
- Carbohydrates: 8 grams
- Sugars: 4 grams
- Fiber: 2 grams

Ingredients Needed:
- ☐ Chicken breasts (1 lb.)

The Dressing:
- ☐ Mayo (1 cup)
- ☐ Lemon juice (2 tbsp.)
- ☐ Sour cream (1 cup)
- ☐ Pepper (1 tsp.)
- ☐ Orange zest (4 tsp.)
- ☐ Salt (.25 tsp.)
- ☐ Orange juice (.33 cup)
- ☐ Chili powder (1 tbsp.)
- ☐ Ground cumin (1 tbsp.)
- ☐ Cayenne pepper (.25 tsp.)
- ☐ Minced garlic (1 clove)

The Salad:
- ☐ Torn lettuce leaves (4 cups)
- ☐ Red onion (1)
- ☐ Tomato (1)
- ☐ Sweet pepper (2 medium - 1 red & 1 green)
- ☐ Shredded cheddar cheese (.5 cup)

Preparation Guidelines:

1. Lightly spritz the grill rack with cooking oil.
2. Remove the bones and skin from the chicken.
3. Grill the prepared chicken, covered, using the medium temperature setting. You can also choose to broil it for five to seven minutes per side (internal temp of 170° Fahrenheit).
4. Grate the orange and whisk the dressing fixings and set it to the side for now.
5. Chop and toss the lettuce, tomato (deseeded), onion, peppers, and cheese in a large mixing container and portion it into eight plates.
6. Cut the chicken into bite-size pieces and toss them over salad with a spritz of salad dressing.

Rodeo King

Servings: 6 | **Difficulty**: Super Easy | **Time**: 30 min

Nutrition per Serving:1 burger no optional garnishes:

- Calories: 768
- Protein: 42 grams
- Fat: 39 grams
- Sat. Fats: 15 grams
- Carbohydrates: 60 grams
- Sugars: 18 grams
- Fiber: 2 grams

Ingredients Needed:

- ☐ Frozen onion rings (12)
- ☐ Ground beef (2 lb.)
- ☐ Garlic salt & black pepper (.25 tsp. of each)
- ☐ Pepper jack cheese (6 slices)
- ☐ Burger buns - toasted (6)
- ☐ BBQ sauce (1 cup)
- ☐ Bacon strips (6 cooked)

Optional Toppings:
- ☐ Leaves of lettuce
- ☐ Dill pickles
- ☐ Sliced tomatoes

Preparation Guidelines:

1. Bake the onion rings according to package directions.
2. Combine the garlic salt, pepper, and beef, shaping it into six ¾-inch-thick patties.
3. Cook the burgers using the medium temperature setting for five to seven minutes per side (160° Fahrenheit internal temp). Don't place the cheese until the burger is about one minute from being done.
4. Prepare the buns with a portion of barbecue sauce, onion rings, bacon, and toppings to your liking.

Dessert

Dutch Apple Pie

Servings: 8 | **Difficulty**: Easy | **Time**: 1 hour

Nutrition per Serving:

- Calories: 494
- Protein: 4 grams
- Fat: 18 grams
- Sat. Fats: 11 grams
- Carbohydrates: 81 grams
- Sugars: 49 grams
- Fibers: 2 grams

Ingredients Needed:

- ☐ Brown sugar (tightly packed - 1 cup)
- ☐ Oatmeal - Quick-cooking (.5 cup)
- ☐ A-P flour (2 cups)
- ☐ Melted butter (.75 cup)

The Filling:
- ☐ Sugar (.66 cup)
- ☐ Cornstarch (3 tbsp.)
- ☐ Water (1.25 cups - cold)
- ☐ Tart apples (4 cups)
- ☐ Vanilla extract (1 tsp.)

Preparation Guidelines:

1. Warm the oven at 350 °Fahrenheit.
2. Combine the flour, oats, brown sugar, and butter, reserving 1.5 cups for garnishing.
3. Create the crust by pressing the rest of the mixture onto the sides and bottom of an ungreased nine-inch pie plate.
4. Mix the cornstarch, sugar, and water until creamy. Wait for it to boil and simmer the mixture until thickened (2 min.). Transfer the pan to a cool burner.
5. Peel, chop, and stir in the apples with the vanilla.
6. Dump the filling into the crust. Crumble the topping over the top.
7. Bake the pie until the filling is bubbly (40-45 min.). Wait for it to cool on a wire rack before serving.

Oreo Cookie Cheesecake

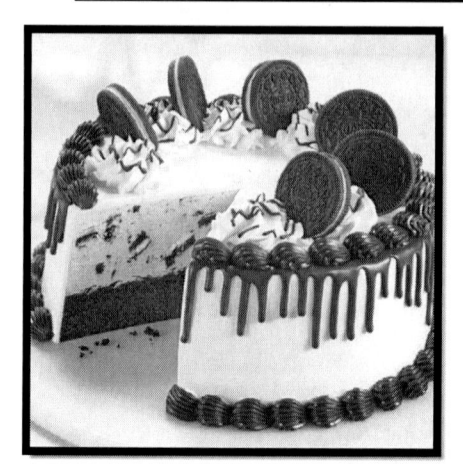

Servings: 8 | **Difficulty**: Easy | **Time**: 40 min + chill time

Nutrition per Serving:

- Calories: 499
- Protein: 7 grams
- Fat: 30 grams
- Sat. Fats: 16 grams
- Carbohydrates: 53 grams
- Fiber: 1 gram
- Sugars: 37 grams

Ingredients Needed:

- ☐ Crushed Oreo cookies (24)
- ☐ Melted butter (6 tbsp.)

The Filling:
- ☐ Unflavored gelatin (1 envelope)
- ☐ Water (.25 cup - cold)
- ☐ Unchilled cream cheese (8 oz. pkg.)
- ☐ Sugar (.5 cup)
- ☐ 2% milk (.75 cup)
- ☐ Whipped topping (1 cup)
- ☐ Oreo cookies (10)
- ☐ Also Needed: 9-inch springform pan

Preparation Guidelines:

1. Lightly grease the pan. Crush and mix the cookies and butter. Press the crust onto the bottom of the pan, and pop it into the fridge until ready to use.
2. Sprinkle the gelatin over cold water and wait for one minute. Heat and stir using the low-temperature setting until it's completely dissolved. Wait for about five minutes.
3. Beat the sugar with the cream cheese until it's smooth, slowly adding the milk. Stir in the gelatin mixture, chopped cookies, and whipped topping. Scoop the mixture over the crust and pop the dish into the fridge (covered) to chill overnight.
4. Serving Time: Use a butter knife to loosen the sides of the cake. If desired, garnish with a few more chopped cookies before serving.

Chapter 3: Cheesecake Factory™ Specialties

Brunch

Cobb Salad Delight

Servings: 6 | **Difficulty**: Very Easy | **Time**: 40 min

Nutrition per Serving:

- Calories: 575
- Protein: 20 grams
- Fat: 52 grams
- Sat. Fats: 8 grams
- Carbohydrates: 10 grams
- Fiber: 5 grams
- Sugars: 3 grams

Ingredients Needed:

- ☐ Red wine vinegar (.25 cup)
- ☐ Lemon juice (.25 cup)
- ☐ Salt (2 tsp.)
- ☐ Garlic (1 small clove)
- ☐ Worcestershire sauce (.75 tsp.)
- ☐ Coarsely ground black pepper (.75 tsp.)
- ☐ Sugar (.25 tsp.)
- ☐ Ground mustard (.25 tsp.)
- ☐ Olive oil (.25 cup)
- ☐ Canola oil (.75 cup)

The Salad:
- ☐ Romaine (6.5 cups)
- ☐ Curly endive (2.5 cups)
- ☐ Watercress - divided (4 oz. bunch)
- ☐ Cooked chicken breasts (2)
- ☐ Tomatoes (2 medium)
- ☐ Ripe avocado (1 medium)
- ☐ Hard-boiled eggs (3 large)
- ☐ Bacon (6 strips - cooked)
- ☐ Crumbled blue/Roquefort cheese (.5 cup)
- ☐ Fresh chives (2 tbsp.)

Preparation Guidelines:

1. Do the prep. Mince the garlic and tear the romaine and endive.
2. Trim the watercress and chop the chicken and tomatoes (deseeded).
3. Peel and chop the avocado and mince the chives. Crumble the cheese and cook the bacon until it's crispy.
4. Prepare a blender by adding the vinegar, salt, juice, garlic, pepper, sugar, mustard, and Worcestershire sauce (up to the line). While processing, slowly pour in both of the oils in a steady stream.
5. Combine and toss the endive, romaine, and half of the watercress into a bowl.
6. Toss the eggs, chicken, avocado, tomatoes, cheese, and bacon over the greens with a sprinkle of chives. Garnish it using the rest of the watercress. Cover and chill until it's serving time.
7. Serve the salad with one cup of dressing over the salad and the balance on the side if desired.

Crispy Crab Cakes

Servings: 8 | **Difficulty**: Easy | **Time**: 20 min

Nutrition per Serving:

- Calories: 282
- Carbohydrates: 7 grams
- Protein: 14 grams
- Fat: 22 grams
- Sat. Fats: 3 grams
- Sugars: 1 gram
- Fiber: 1 gram

Ingredients Needed:

- ☐ Crabmeat (1 lb. fresh/canned - cartilage removed & flaked)
- ☐ Soft breadcrumbs (2-2.5 cups)
- ☐ Whisked egg (1 large)
- ☐ Mayonnaise (.75 cup)
- ☐ Chopped veggies (.33 cup each)
    - ☐ Celery
    - ☐ Onion
    - ☐ Green Pepper
- ☐ Seafood seasoning (1 tbsp.)
- ☐ Fresh parsley (1 tbsp.)
- ☐ Black pepper (.25 tsp.)
- ☐ Worcestershire sauce (1 tsp.)
- ☐ Lemon juice (2 tsp.)
- ☐ Hot pepper sauce (1/8 tsp.)
- ☐ Prepared mustard (1 tsp.)

Optional Ingredients:
- ☐ Vegetable oil (2-4 tbsp.)
- ☐ Lemon wedges

Preparation Guidelines:

1. Chop the veggies and combine with the rest of the fixings (crab, egg, breadcrumbs, mayo, seasonings). Shape the mixture into eight patties.
2. Cook the patties for four minutes per side in an oven-proof skillet using enough oil to cover the pan.
3. Serve it with a wedge of lime if desired.

Lunch or Dinner

Cuban Sandwich Specialty

Servings: 4 | **Difficulty**: Easy | **Time**: 25 min

Nutrition per Serving:
- Calories: 545
- Carbohydrates: 41 grams
- Protein: 33 grams
- Fat: 27 grams
- Sat. Fats: 12 grams
- Sugars: 4 grams
- Fiber: 2 grams

Ingredients Needed:
- ☐ Garlic (2 cloves)
- ☐ Olive oil (.5 tsp.)
- ☐ Red-fat mayonnaise (.5 cup)
- ☐ Artisan bread (8 slices)
- ☐ Deli ham (4 slices)
- ☐ Deli smoked turkey (8 thick slices)
- ☐ Swiss cheese (8 slices)
- ☐ Baby spinach (1 cup)
- ☐ Dill pickle (12 slices)

Preparation Guidelines:
1. Mince and add the garlic into a skillet with the oil to sauté using the med-high heat until tender. Cool for a few minutes.
2. Stir the cooled garlic into the mayo and spread it over the bread slices.
3. Layer four slices of bread with the ham, turkey, cheese, spinach, and pickles. Close and cook on a panini maker or indoor grill until browned and the cheese is melted (2-3 min.).

Fish & Chips

Servings: 4 | **Difficulty**: Very easy | **Time**: 30 min

Nutrition per Serving - 1 fillet and ¾ cup of fries:

- Calories: 416
- Carbohydrates: 26 grams
- Protein: 32 grams
- Fat: 19 grams
- Sat. Fats: 4 grams
- Fiber: 2 grams
- Sugars: 2 grams

Ingredients Needed:

- ☐ Frozen steak fries (4 cups)
- ☐ Salmon fillets (4 @ 6 ounces each)
- ☐ Prepared horseradish (1-2 tbsp.)
- ☐ Dijon-style mustard (1 tsp.)
- ☐ Worcestershire sauce (1 tbsp.)
- ☐ Parmesan cheese (1 tbsp. - grated)
- ☐ Salt (.25 tsp.)
- ☐ Panko breadcrumbs (.5 cup)
- ☐ Cooking oil spray (as needed)

Preparation Guidelines:

1. Warm the oven at 450° Fahrenheit. Adjust the rack to the lowest setting.
2. Arrange the fries on a baking sheet (one layer). Set the timer to bake until they are as you like them (15-20 min.).
3. Lightly spritz a baking pan using cooking oil. Arrange the salmon on it and set it aside.
4. Mix the horseradish, cheese, Worcestershire sauce, salt, and mustard. Stir in the breadcrumbs. Press the coating over each of the fillets. Spritz the tops using cooking oil spray.
5. Adjust the rack to the middle setting. Place the tray on the oven rack and set the timer to bake the fish for ten minutes. Serve when it's ready (easily flakes) with the fries.

Fish Tacos

Servings: 4 | **Difficulty**: Very Easy | **Time**: 30 min

Nutrition per Serving:

- Calories: 321
- Protein: 34 grams
- Fat: 10 grams
- Sat. Fats: 5 grams
- Carbohydrates: 29 grams
- Fiber: 4 grams
- Sugars: 5 grams

Ingredients Needed:

- ☐ Fat-free mayonnaise (.5 cup)
- ☐ Lime juice (1 tbsp.)
- ☐ Fat-free milk (2 tsp.)
- ☐ Large egg (1)
- ☐ Water (1 tsp.)
- ☐ Breadcrumbs (.33 cup)
- ☐ Lemon-pepper seasoning - salt-free (2 tbsp.)
- ☐ Cod/Mahi Mahi fillets - 1-inch strips (1 lb.)
- ☐ Corn tortillas - warmed (4 @ 6-inch each)

The Toppings:
- ☐ Coleslaw mix (1 cup)
- ☐ Chopped tomatoes (2 medium)
- ☐ Mexican cheese blend - shredded & reduced-fat (1 cup)
- ☐ Freshly minced cilantro (1 tbsp.)

Preparation Guidelines:

1. Prepare the sauce. Whisk the lime juice, mayo, and milk in a mixing container. Pop it in the fridge until it's time to eat.
2. Whisk the egg and water.
3. In a separate shallow container, toss the lemon pepper with the breadcrumbs.
4. Dip fish in the egg mixture, crumb mixture, and pat them to help the coating stick.
5. Prepare a skillet using the med-high temperature setting. Add the fish to cook for two to four minutes per side or until they're nicely browned, and fish just begins to flake easily with a fork.
6. Enjoy it in tortillas with delicious toppings and a sauce of your liking.

Goat Cheese & Beet Salad

Servings: 12 | **Difficulty**: Easy | **Time**: 1.2 hours

Nutrition per Serving:

- Calories: 125
- Fat: 9 grams
- Sat. Fats: 2 grams
- Protein: 4 grams
- Carbohydrates: 10 grams
- Fiber: 2 grams
- Sugars: 6 grams

Ingredients Needed:

- [ ] Fresh beets (3 medium/1 lb.)
- [ ] Orange zest (1 tsp.)
- [ ] Honey (2 tsp.)
- [ ] Dijon-style mustard (1 tsp.)
- [ ] White wine vinegar (1 tbsp.)
- [ ] Orange juice (2 tbsp.)
- [ ] Olive oil (3 tbsp.)
- [ ] Black pepper (.25 tsp.)
- [ ] Salt (.5 tsp.)
- [ ] Freshly minced tarragon - divided (3 tbsp.)
- [ ] Fresh baby spinach (6 oz. pkg.)
- [ ] Torn mixed salad greens (4 cups)
- [ ] Navel oranges (2 medium)
- [ ] Crumbled goat cheese (4 oz.)
- [ ] Toasted - chopped walnuts (.5 cup)

Preparation Guidelines:

1. Set the oven temperature at 425° Fahrenheit.
2. Scrub the beets and trim tops to one inch and wrap them in foil. Put them on a baking tray to cook for 50-60 minutes. Discard the foil and cool thoroughly. Peel the beets and cut into wedges.
3. Peel and section the oranges. Zest the peels. Whisk the vinegar, oil, orange zest, orange juice, honey, salt, pepper, mustard until blended.
4. Stir in one tablespoon of tarragon. Combine the spinach, salad greens, and rest of the tarragon. Drizzle with vinaigrette and toss gently to coat.
5. Transfer to a platter or divide among 12 salad plates. Top with orange sections and beets; sprinkle with cheese and walnuts. Serve promptly.

Merlot Filet Mignon

Servings: 2 | **Difficulty**: Super Easy | **Time**: 20 min

Nutrition per Serving 1 steak + 2 tbsp. sauce:

- Calories: 690
- Carbohydrates: 4 grams
- Protein: 49 grams
- Fat: 43 grams
- Sat. Fats: 20 grams
- Sugars: 1 gram
- Fiber: 0 grams

Ingredients Needed:
- ☐ Beef tenderloin steaks (2 - 8 oz. each)
- ☐ Butter (3 tbsp. - divided)
- ☐ Olive oil (1 tbsp.)
- ☐ Merlot (1 cup)
- ☐ Heavy whipping cream (2 tbsp.)
- ☐ Salt (1/8 tsp.)

Preparation Guidelines:

1. Prepare a skillet using the medium temperature setting to cook the steaks in one tablespoon butter and the olive oil for four to six minutes per side. The desired doneness for medium-rare is 135° Fahrenheit; medium, 140° Fahrenheit; medium-well, 145° Fahrenheit (internal temperature). Remove the steaks from the pan and keep warm.
2. In the same skillet, pour in the wine, stirring to loosen the browned bits from the pan. Wait for it to boil, and cook until the juices are reduced to about ¼ of a cup. Add the cream, salt, and rest of the butter. Cook and stir until slightly thickened, and butter is melted (1-2 min.). Relax and serve with the steaks.

Pasta Da Vinci

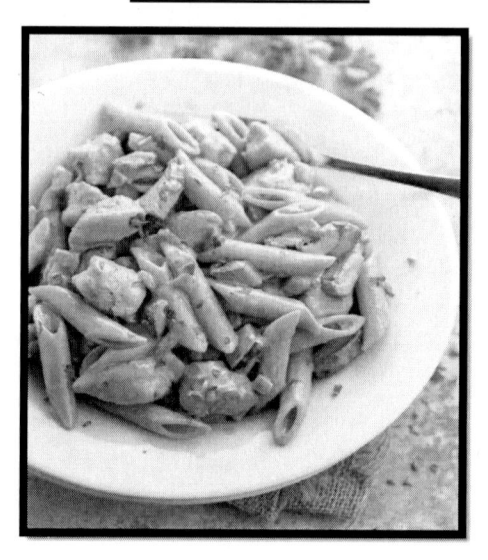

Servings: 6 | **Difficulty**: Easy | **Time**: 45 min

Nutrition per Serving:

- Calories: 712
- Carbohydrates: 66 grams
- Protein: 32 grams
- Fat: 32 grams
- Sat. Fats: 18 grams
- Sugars: 5 grams
- Fiber: 4 grams

Ingredients Needed:

- [ ] Penne pasta (1 lb.)
- [ ] Butter - divided (4 tbsp.)
- [ ] Chicken breast (1 lb. into 1-inch chunks)
- [ ] Black pepper (.25 tsp.)
- [ ] Kosher salt (.5 tsp.)
- [ ] Shiitake/crimini mushrooms (1 lb. sliced)
- [ ] Red onion (1 chopped)
- [ ] Garlic cloves (2)
- [ ] Madeira wine (1 cup)
- [ ] Heavy cream (.5 cup)
- [ ] Sour cream (.5 cup)
- [ ] Chicken broth (1 cup)
- [ ] Parmesan cheese (.5 cup)
- [ ] Also Needed: Cast-iron skillet

Preparation Guidelines:

1. Cook the pasta for one minute using the package directions.
2. Melt one tablespoon of butter in the skillet. Add the chicken and cook using the med-high temperature setting for five to seven minutes. Set it aside with the pasta fixings.
3. Add butter (1 tbsp.) to melt and add the mushrooms to sauté for five to seven minutes. Add another tablespoon of butter and add the onions, sautéing for another five minutes or so, using the med-low setting.
4. Mince and mix in the garlic to sauté for one minute. Pour in the wine and chicken broth to simmer for 10-12 minutes until it's reduced (by ¾ of the liquids).
5. Mix in the heavy cream, sour cream, last of the butter (1 tbsp.), and parmesan. Whisk well and add the rest of the fixings.
6. Sprinkle it with more parmesan and serve.

Southern-Fried Catfish

Servings: 4 | **Difficulty**: Easy | **Time**: 20 min

Nutrition per Serving:

- Calories: 475
- Carbohydrates: 10 grams
- Protein: 29 grams
- Fat: 34 grams
- Sat. Fats: 5 grams
- Sugars: 0 grams
- Fiber: 1 gram

Ingredients Needed:

- ☐ Eggs (2)
- ☐ Carbonated water (2 tbsp.)
- ☐ Pancake mix (1 cup)
- ☐ Black pepper (.25 tsp.)
- ☐ Seasoned salt (.5 tsp.)
- ☐ Catfish fillets (4 @ 6 oz. each)
- ☐ For Frying: Oil as needed

Preparation Guidelines:

1. Whisk the eggs and water in a mixing container.
2. In another shallow dish, whisk the pancake mix, seasoned salt, and pepper. Dip fillets in the egg mixture and coat with seasoned pancake mix.
3. In an electric skillet, warm the oil at 375° Fahrenheit. Fry the fillets for two to three minutes until nicely browned.
4. Press them into paper towels to remove the excess grease before serving.

The Everything Pizza

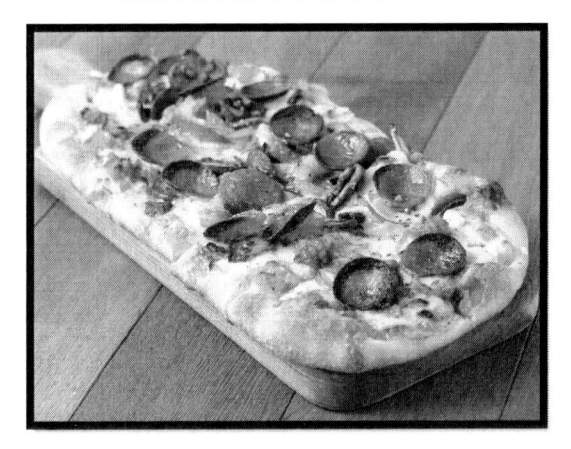

Servings: 8 slices | **Difficulty**: Medium | **Time**: 60 min

Nutrition per Serving:
- Calories: 596
- Carbohydrates: 41 grams
- Protein: 33 grams
- Fat: 34 grams
- Sat. Fats: 16 grams
- Sugars: 3 grams
- Fiber: 3 grams

Ingredients Needed:
- ☐ Active dry yeast (.25 oz. pkg.)
- ☐ Warm water - 110° Fahrenheit to 115° Fahrenheit (.5 cup)
- ☐ Melted & cooled butter (.5 cup)
- ☐ Large eggs (3)
- ☐ Grated parmesan cheese (.25 cup)
- ☐ Bread flour (3-3.5 cups)
- ☐ Salt (1 tsp.)
- ☐ Yellow cornmeal (2 tbsp.)
- ☐ Ground beef (.5 lb.)
- ☐ Bulk Italian sausage (.5 lb.)
- ☐ Onion (1 small)

- ☐ Pizza sauce (2 - 8 oz. cans)
- ☐ Sliced mushrooms (4.5 oz. jar)
- ☐ Sliced pepperoni (3 oz. pkg.)
- ☐ Cubed deli ham (.5 lb.)
- ☐ Pitted green olives (.5 cup)
- ☐ Ripe black olives (4.25 oz. can)
- ☐ Part-skim mozzarella cheese (1.5 cups - shredded)
- ☐ Shredded parmesan cheese (.5 cup)
- ☐ Also Needed: 12-inch deep cast-iron skillet or another oven-proof pan (+) another skillet for the meat

Preparation Guidelines:

1. Chop the onion. Drain and chop the olives, and drain the sliced mushrooms.
2. Mix the warm water and yeast and wait for it to dissolve.
3. Combine the yeast mixture, salt, parmesan eggs, butter, and two cups of flour. Beat using the medium speed of a mixer until it's creamy smooth. Mix in more flour to create a soft dough.
4. Flip the dough out onto a floured cutting board and knead six to eight minutes until it's smooth and elastic. Place it in a greased mixing container turning once to form a layer of oil on its top. Cover the dish with a layer of plastic wrap. Place it in a warm space to rise for about one hour until it has doubled in size.
5. Punch the dough back down and wait for about five minutes.
6. Warm the oven setting to 400° Fahrenheit. Grease the skillet and dust it using the cornmeal. Press the prepared dough into the pan.
7. Use another skillet for cooking the onion, sausage, and beef (8-10 min.) and drain.
8. Spread the sauce over the dough (leave 1-inch edges), sprinkle with the cooked meat, mushrooms, ham, pepperoni, olives, and all of the cheese.
9. Bake the pizza for 30 to 35 minutes until the cheese is brown and serve.

White Chicken Chili

Servings: 6 | **Difficulty**: Very Easy | **Time**: 30 min

Nutrition per Serving:

- Calories: 228
- Protein: 22 grams
- Fat: 5 grams
- Sat. Fats: 1 gram
- Carbohydrates: 23 grams
- Fiber: 6 grams
- Sugars: 1 gram

Ingredients Needed:

- ☐ Lean ground chicken (1 lb.)
- ☐ Onion (1 medium)
- ☐ Green chiles (4 oz. can)
- ☐ Cannellini beans (2 - 15 oz. cans)
- ☐ Black pepper (.25 tsp.)
- ☐ Dried oregano (.5 tsp.)
- ☐ Ground cumin (1 tsp.)
- ☐ Reduced-sodium chicken broth (14.5 oz.)

Optional Garnishes:
- ☐ Sour cream - low-fat
- ☐ Freshly chopped cilantro
- ☐ Shredded cheddar cheese

Preparation Guidelines:

1. Wash the beans in a colander and drain. Chop the onion and chilies.
2. Cook the chicken and onion using the med-high temperature setting until the chicken is no longer pink (6-8 min.), breaking it up as it cooks.
3. Pour one can of beans in a small bowl and slightly mash. Stir the mashed beans, with the remaining can of beans, seasonings, chiles, and broth into chicken mixture. Once boiling, lower the temperature setting and simmer, covered (12-15 min.).
4. Serve with toppings to your liking.
5. Notes: Freeze cooked and cooled chili in freezer containers.
6. To use, partially thaw in the fridge overnight.
7. Thoroughly warm in a saucepan, stirring occasionally, and adding additional broth if needed.

Dessert

Caramel Pecan Turtle Cheesecake

Servings: 8 | **Difficulty**: Easy | **Time**: 25 min

Nutrition per Serving:
- Calories: 585
- Carbohydrates: 53 grams
- Protein: 7 grams
- Fat: 40 grams
- Sat. Fats: 20 grams
- Sugars: 23 grams

Ingredients Needed:
- ☐ New York-style cheesecake (Frozen - thawed 30 oz. cake)
- ☐ Heavy whipping cream (.5 cup - divided)
- ☐ Semi-sweet chocolate chips (.5 cup)
- ☐ Toasted chopped pecans (3 tbsp.)
- ☐ Packed brown sugar (.5 cup + 2 tbsp.)
- ☐ Cubed butter (.25 cup)
- ☐ Light corn syrup (1 tbsp.)

Preparation Guidelines:
1. Thaw and place the cheesecake on a serving platter cake tray.
2. Toss the chocolate chips in a mixing container.
3. Warm ¼ cup of cream. Once it is boiling, mix it with the chocolate and stir until it's creamy. Cool slightly and dump it over cheesecake with a sprinkle with pecans. Pop it into the fridge to set.
4. Prepare a saucepan to melt the butter, brown sugar, and corn syrup. Once boiling, lower the temperature setting and simmer until the sugar is dissolved. Stir in the remainder of the cream. Once it's hot, serve it over the cheesecake.

Pumpkin Cheesecake

Servings: 24 | **Difficulty**: Medium | **Time**: 1 hour

Nutrition per Serving:
- Calories: 276
- Carbohydrates: 20 grams
- Protein: 5 grams
- Fat: 20 grams
- Sat. Fats: 11 grams
- Sugars: 13 grams
- Fiber: 1 gram

Ingredients Needed:
- [ ] Crushed gingersnaps (1.5 cups/approx 30 cookies)
- [ ] Melted butter (.25 cup)
- [ ] Softened cream cheese (5 - 8 oz. pkg.)
- [ ] Sugar (1 cup)
- [ ] Solid-pack pumpkin (15 oz. can)
- [ ] Ground cinnamon (1 tsp.)
- [ ] Whisked unchilled eggs (5 large)
- [ ] Vanilla extract (1 tsp.)
- [ ] Maple syrup
- [ ] Ground nutmeg (1-2 pinches)
- [ ] Optional: Sweetened whipped cream
- [ ] Also Needed: 13x9-inch baking dish

Preparation Guidelines:

1. Warm the oven temperature at 350° Fahrenheit.
2. Crush and combine the gingersnap crumbs and butter. Press onto the bottom of a greased dish and set it to the side for now.
3. Mix the sugar and cream cheese until smooth. Fold in the vanilla, pumpkin, and cinnamon. Whisk and add the eggs, using the low setting of an electric mixer just until combined. Pour over the crust and sprinkle it with nutmeg.
4. Bake the pie for 40 to 45 minutes or until the center is almost set. Let it rest on a wire rack for ten minutes. Gently loosen the edge of the baking dish to loosen the cake's edges. Cool one more hour or refrigerate overnight for the best results.
5. Slice the cake and serve with syrup and sweetened whipped cream.

Chapter 4: Taco Bell™ Specialties

Breakfast

AM Crunchwrap

Servings: 2 | **Difficulty**: Very Easy | **Time**: 30 min

Nutrition per Serving:

- Calories: 255
- Carbohydrates: 16 grams
- Protein: 15 grams
- Fat: 14 grams
- Sat. Fats: 6 grams
- Sugars: 2 grams
- Fiber: 1 gram

Ingredients Needed:

- ☐ Flour tortillas (2 large)
- ☐ Whisked eggs (3-4) + Milk (1 tbsp.)
- ☐ Shredded sharp cheddar cheese (2-4 tbsp.)
- ☐ Shredded hash browns (heaping .5 cup)
- ☐ Hot sauce - mild - your choice (4 tbsp.)
- ☐ Bacon (4 crispy)
- ☐ Cooking oil spray
- ☐ Taco Bell sauce

Preparation Guidelines:

1. Lightly spritz a skillet using cooking oil spray and warm using the medium temperature setting.
2. Whisk and add the eggs, salt, and pepper into a skillet. Whisk until they are fluffy and set them aside.
3. Warm a skillet and heat the tortillas for about half of a minute. Prepare and close them, placing them in a skillet to cook for about 30 to 40 seconds using the medium temperature setting.
4. Serve with sauce as desired.

Cinnabon Delights

Servings: 24 | **Difficulty:** Easy | **Time**: 30 min

Nutrition per Serving:
- Calories: 62.1
- Protein: 0.1 grams
- Fat Content: 2.3 grams
- Sat. Fats: 1.4 grams
- Carbohydrates: 10.7 grams
- Fiber: 0.2 grams
- Sugars: 7.8 grams

Ingredients Needed:
- ☐ Pillsbury™ refrigerated cinnamon rolls with icing (24 oz. can)
- ☐ Cinnamon (2 tsp.)
- ☐ Granulated sugar (.75 cup)
- ☐ Butter (.25 cup)
- ☐ Warmed caramel ice cream topping (.25 cup)
- ☐ Betty Crocker™ Rich & Creamy white frosting (.25 cup)

Preparation Guidelines:
1. Heat the oven at 350° Fahrenheit. Prepare a baking tray using a layer of parchment baking paper. Open the rolls and slice each one into three pieces. Roll each one into a ball.
2. Add the butter to a small microwave-safe dish to melt. Whisk the sugar and cinnamon in another bowl.
3. Roll the dough balls through the butter, then the cinnamon and sugar. Arrange them on the baking tin. Bake them until nicely browned (ten min.) and cool for another ten minutes.
4. Warm the frosting for about ten seconds in the microwave to soften it slightly for piping. Scoop the filling into the piping bag.
5. Squirt in the frosting into the ball until it puffs. Garnish them using the sauce and serve.

Dressed Egg Taco

Servings: 8 | **Difficulty**: Easy | **Time**: 25 min

Nutrition per Serving:

- Calories: 291
- Protein: 13 grams
- Fat: 16 grams
- Sat. Fats: 6 grams
- Carbohydrates: 22 grams
- Sugars: 1 gram
- Fiber: 3 grams

Ingredients Needed:

- ☐ Black beans (.33 cup)
- ☐ Pico de Gallo (.33 cup)
- ☐ Cubed avocado (.33 cup)
- ☐ Lime juice (1 tbsp.)
- ☐ Frozen - thawed potatoes (1 cup)
- ☐ Bulk pork sausage (.5 lb)
- ☐ Eggs (6 large)
- ☐ 2% milk (2 tbsp.)
- ☐ Monterey Jack shredded cheese (.5 cup)
- ☐ Warmed flour tortillas (8 @ 6-inches)

Optional Fixings:
- ☐ Pico de Gallo
- ☐ Sour cream
- ☐ Freshly chopped cilantro

Preparation Guidelines:

1. Rinse and drain the beans.
2. Gently mix the avocado, beans, pico de gallo, and lime juice.
3. In a large cast-iron or another heavy skillet, cook the potatoes and crumbled sausage using the medium temperature setting until the sausage is no longer pink (6-8 min.).
4. Whisk the eggs and milk. Pour them into the skillet, stirring over medium heat until the eggs are thickened, and no liquid egg remains.
5. Stir in the cheese.
6. Spoon the egg mixture into each of the tortillas, and top with the bean mixture. Garnish them to your liking.

Lunch

Delicious Tacos

Servings: 12 | **Difficulty**: Very Easy | **Time**: 30 min

Nutrition per Serving:

- Calories: 236
- Protein: 12 grams
- Fat: 15 grams
- Sat. Fats: 6 grams
- Carbohydrates: 10 grams
- Fiber: 1 gram
- Sugars: 1 gram

Ingredients Needed:
- ☐ Ground chuck (1.33 lb.)
- ☐ Golden Masa Harina corn flour - ex. Bob's Red Mill (1.5 tbsp.)
- ☐ Chili powder (4.5 tsp.)
- ☐ Sugar (.25 tsp.)
- ☐ Ground cumin (.25 tsp.)
- ☐ Dried minced onion (1 tsp.)

Spices @.5 tsp.
- ☐ Onion powder
- ☐ Seasoning salt
- ☐ Garlic powder
- ☐ Paprika
- ☐ Garlic salt
- ☐ Beef bouillon powder

To Serve:
- ☐ Taco shells (12)
- ☐ Shredded Iceberg lettuce (half of 1 head)
- ☐ Diced Roma tomatoes (2)
- ☐ Shredded cheddar cheese (1 cup)
- ☐ Optional: Sour cream

Preparation Guidelines:

1. Combine all of the 'beef filling' fixings except for the meat. Combine the spice mix - blending thoroughly.
2. Cook the beef in a skillet until browned. Transfer it from the burner and dump the meat into a strainer to rinse with hot water.
3. Toss the beef into the pan and stir in the spice mix with water (.75-1 cup). Simmer using the med-low temperature setting to cook away most of the liquids (20 min.)
4. Prepare the tacos. Pop the shells into a 350° Fahrenheit oven for 7-10 minutes.
5. Assemble them with the meat, lettuce, tomatoes, sour cream, and cheese to your liking.
6. Serve them promptly.

Dinner

Chalupa Supreme

Servings: 6 | **Difficulty**: Simple | **Time**: 35 min

Nutrition per Serving:

- Calories: 206
- Carbohydrates: 17 grams
- Protein: 19 grams
- Fat: 6 grams
- Sat. Fats: 2 grams
- Sugars: 3 grams
- Fiber: 3 grams

Ingredients Needed:

- ☐ Corn tortillas (6 @ 6-inches)
- ☐ Olive oil (2 tsp.)
- ☐ Shredded part-skim mozzarella cheese (.75 cup)
- ☐ Cooked chicken breast (2 cups)
- ☐ Diced tomatoes with green chiles (14.5 oz. can - undrained)
- ☐ Ground cumin (1 tsp.)
- ☐ Garlic powder (1 tsp.)
- ☐ Black pepper and salt (.25 tsp. of each)
- ☐ Onion powder (1 tsp.)
- ☐ Finely shredded cabbage (.5 cup)

Preparation Guidelines:

1. Warm the oven in advance at 350 °Fahrenheit. Arrange the tortillas on an ungreased baking sheet. Brush them using a bit of oil and a sprinkle of cheese.
2. Chop and toss the chicken, tomatoes, and seasonings in a large skillet. Simmer and stir using the medium temperature setting (6-8 min.) or until most of the liquid is evaporated.
3. Spoon the delicious mixture over the tortillas.
4. Bake for 15-18 minutes until the tortillas are crisp and cheese is melted. Garnish with the cabbage.

Grilled Steak Soft Tacos

Servings: 6 | **Difficulty**: Easy | **Time**: 30 min

Nutrition per Serving:

- Calories: 329
- Protein: 27 grams
- Fat: 12 grams
- Sat. Fats: 4 grams
- Carbohydrates: 29 grams
- Sugars: 3 grams
- Fiber: 5 grams

Ingredients Needed:

The Salsa:
- ☐ Large tomatoes (2)
- ☐ Red onion (.5 cup)
- ☐ Lime juice (.25 cup)
- ☐ Jalapeno pepper (1)
- ☐ Fresh cilantro (3 tbsp.)
- ☐ Salt - divided (.75 tsp.)
- ☐ Ground cumin - divided (2 tsp.)
- ☐ Beef flank steak (approx. 1.5 lb.)
- ☐ Canola oil (1 tbsp.)
- ☐ Whole wheat tortillas (6 warmed - 8-inches)
- ☐ Onion (1 large - sliced)
- ☐ Optional: Lime wedges & sliced avocado

Preparation Guidelines:

1. Deseed and chop the tomatoes and jalapeno. Dice the onion and cilantro.
2. Prepare the salsa by combining the first five fixings (before the line). Stir in one teaspoon cumin and ¼ teaspoon salt. Set it to the side for now.
3. Sprinkle the steak using the rest of the salt and cumin.
4. Grill using the medium temperature setting (with a lid on) until the meat is as you like it (med-rare, on an instant-read thermometer, is about 135 °Fahrenheit), or 6-8 minutes. Let the cooked meat stand for five minutes before slicing.
5. Warm the oil in a skillet using the med-high temperature setting and sauté them until the onion is crisp-tender.
6. Slice steak thinly across the grain and serve on tortillas with onion and salsa.
7. If desired, serve with avocado and lime wedges.

XXL Grilled Stuffed Burrito

Servings: 6 | **Difficulty**: Very Easy| **Time**: 25 min

Nutrition per Serving - no toppings calculated:

- Calories: 452
- Protein: 21 grams
- Fat: 13 grams
- Sat. Fats: 5 grams
- Carbohydrates: 56 grams
- Sugars: 4 grams
- Fiber: 9 grams

Ingredients Needed:

- ☐ Black beans (.75 cup)
- ☐ Whole grain rice medley - ex. Santa Fe ready-to-serve (8.5 oz. pkg.)
- ☐ 90% Lean ground beef (.5 lb.)
- ☐ Frozen corn (.75 cup)
- ☐ Salsa of choice (12 oz. jar.)
- ☐ Velvetta thinly sliced processed cheese (4 oz.)
- ☐ 10-inch flour tortillas (6 - warmed)

Optional Toppings:
- ☐ Torn lettuce leaves
- ☐ Sour cream
- ☐ Shredded Mexican cheese blend
- ☐ Chopped sweet red pepper & onions
- ☐ Also Needed: 4-qt. microwave-safe dish

Preparation Guidelines:

1. Measure and add the beans into a colander. Thoroughly rinse and drain them.
2. Warm the rice and crumble beef into the baking dish. Thaw and add in the corn and beans.
3. Microwave, covered, using the high-temperature setting until the beef is no longer pink (4-5 min.) and drain.
4. Stir in salsa and cheese and microwave until the cheese is melted (2-3 min.). Fold in rice.
5. Spoon ¾ cup of the beef mixture into the center of each tortilla. Add additional ingredients as desired.
6. Fold the bottom and sides of the tortilla over filling and roll it up. Enjoy them at dinner or anytime!

Desserts

TB Baja Blast Freeze

Servings: 1 | **Difficulty**: Easy | **Time**: 6 min

Nutrition per Serving:

- Calories: 414
- Carbohydrates: 106 grams
- Protein: 0 grams
- Fat: 0 grams
- Sat. Fats: 0 grams
- Sugars: 103 grams
- Fiber: 0 grams

Ingredients Needed:

- ☐ Mountain Dew (8 oz.)
- ☐ Powerade Berry Blast (3 oz.)
- ☐ Ice (6 cubes/as desired)

Preparation Guidelines:

1. Toss each of the fixings into a blender.
2. Pulse until the ice is crushed and serve promptly for the best results.

Taco Bell Crispitos

Servings: 6 | **Difficulty**: Very Easy | **Time**: 20 min

Nutrition per Serving:

- Calories: 443
- Protein: 8 grams
- Fat: 15 grams
- Sat. Fats: 9 grams
- Carbohydrates: 67 grams
- Sugars: 21 grams
- Fiber: 2 grams

Ingredients Needed:

- ☐ Cinnamon (⅛ cup)
- ☐ Sugar (.5 cup)
- ☐ Tortillas (10)
- ☐ To Fry: Vegetable oil

Preparation Guidelines:

1. Combine the sugar and cinnamon.
2. Warm a skillet/dutch oven (medium-high/approx. 350° Fahrenheit). Don't let it get "smoking" hot.
3. Use a sharp knife to quarter the tortillas. Deep-fry them two to four at a time for about half a minute per side. Place them onto a paper-lined wire rack to cool.
4. While they are draining, sprinkle them using the sugar-cinnamon mixture and serve.

Chapter 5: Olive Garden™ Specialties

Brunch

Eggplant Parmigiana

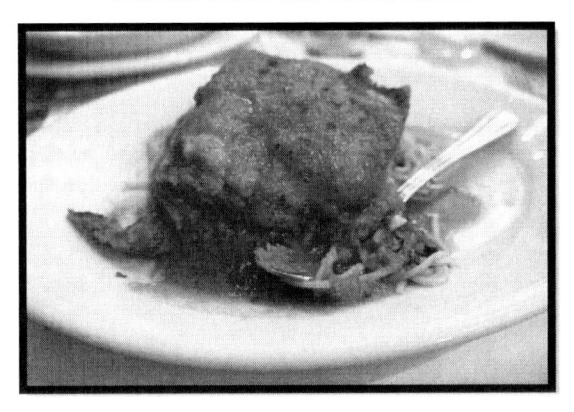

Servings: 8 | **Difficulty**: Medium | **Time**: 1 hour min

Nutrition per Serving:

- Calories: 305
- Protein: 18 grams
- Fat: 12 grams
- Sat. Fats: 5 grams
- Carbohydrates: 32 grams
- Sugars: 12 grams
- Fibers: 9 grams

Ingredients Needed:

- ☐ Large eggs (3)
- ☐ Panko breadcrumbs (2.5 cups)
- ☐ Eggplants (3 medium @ ¼ inch slices)
- ☐ Jars of mushrooms (2 @ 4.5 oz. each)
- ☐ Dried basil (.5 tsp.)
- ☐ Dried oregano (⅛ tsp.)
- ☐ Grated parmesan cheese (.5 cup)
- ☐ Part-skim mozzarella cheese (2 cups - shredded)
- ☐ spaghetti sauce (28 oz. jar)
- ☐ Also Needed: 13x9-inch baking dish

Preparation Guidelines:

1. Drain and slice the mushrooms.
2. Warm the oven to reach 350 °Fahrenheit. Lightly spritz a baking sheet (s) with cooking oil.
3. Place eggs and breadcrumbs into two shallow bowls.
4. Dip the eggplant in the whisked eggs and coat in the crumbs.
5. Arrange them on the prepared trays.
6. Bake for 15-20 minutes, turning once.
7. Drain the mushrooms and mix with the basil and oregano.
8. In another mixing bowl, combine both types of cheese.
9. Spread ½ cup of sauce into the prepared baking dish. Layer the fixings using 1/3 portions of each of the mushroom mixture and eggplant, 3/4 cup of sauce, and 1/3 of the cheese mixture. Continue the process in two more layers.
10. Leave the lid off and bake it at 350 °Fahrenheit for 25-30 minutes or until the cheese is melted.

Shrimp & Chicken Carbonara

Servings: 6 | **Difficulty**: Medium | **Time**: 1 hour

Nutrition per Serving:

- Calories: 956.4
- Protein: 50.7 grams
- Fat: 54 grams
- Sat. Fats: 23.5 grams
- Carbohydrates: 66.3 grams
- Sugars: 3.8 grams
- Fiber: 3.7 grams

Ingredients Needed:

- ☐ Jumbo shrimp (1 lb.)
- ☐ Smoked bacon (8 slices)
- ☐ Chicken breast halves (1 lb.)
- ☐ Olive oil - divided (4 tbsp.)
- ☐ Garlic - divided (3 tbsp.)
- ☐ Italian seasoning (2 tbsp.)
- ☐ Linguine pasta (16 oz. pkg.)
- ☐ Onion (1)
- ☐ Heavy whipping cream (1.5 cups)
- ☐ Egg yolks (4)
- ☐ Parmesan cheese (1.5 cups - grated)
- ☐ Freshly cracked black pepper and salt (1 pinch/as desired)
- ☐ Sauvignon Blanc wine (.25 cup)

Preparation Guidelines:

1. Peel and devein the shrimp and dice the bacon. Discard the bones and skin from the chicken. Chop it into bite-sized pieces.
2. Prepare a skillet to warm one tablespoon of oil using the med-high temperature setting. Cook and stir the chicken with one tablespoon of minced garlic and one tablespoon of Italian seasoning (6-8 min.). Dump the chicken into a bowl for now.
3. Warm one tablespoon garlic and one tablespoon olive oil in the same skillet. Fry the shrimp until it's a pinkish-red (6-8 min.). Place it with the chicken.
4. Add water to a large pot and wait for it to boil. Add the rest of the oil (two tablespoons). Cook the linguine until it's al dente (10-12 min.). Dump it into a colander to drain.
5. Toss the bacon into the pan to cook until it's just crispy, not crunchy (6 min.). Drain on two paper towels. Dice and sauté the onion in the bacon grease until translucent (approx. 5 min.).
6. While the onion is sauteing, mix the cream, parmesan cheese, egg yolks, salt, pepper, and rest of the Italian seasoning in a mixing bowl.
7. Measure and add the wine into the pan with the onions. Increase the temperature setting and wait for it to boil. Simmer it until the wine is mostly evaporated (about 2 min.). Add the creamy egg mixture and reduce heat. Simmer until sauce begins to thicken (3-5 min.). Add the chicken and shrimp; mix to coat. Serve on top of a platter of pasta.

Lunch

Chicken & Gnocchi Soup

Servings: 2 quarts/8 portions | **Difficulty**: Easy | **Time**: 40 min

Nutrition per Serving:

- Calories: 482
- Protein: 21 grams
- Fat: 28 grams
- Sat. Fats: 17 grams
- Carbohydrates: 36 grams
- Sugars: 10 grams
- Fiber: 2 grams

Ingredients Needed:

- ☐ Chicken breasts (1 lb.)
- ☐ Butter - divided (.33 cup)
- ☐ Small onion (1)
- ☐ Carrot (1 medium)
- ☐ Celery (1 rib)
- ☐ Garlic (2 cloves)
- ☐ All-purpose flour (.33 cup)
- ☐ Heavy whipping cream (1.5 cups)
- ☐ 2% milk (3.5 cups)
- ☐ Chicken bouillon granules (1 tbsp.)
- ☐ Coarsely ground pepper (.25 tsp.)
- ☐ Potato gnocchi (16 oz. pkg.)
- ☐ Fresh spinach (.5 cup)

Preparation Guidelines:

1. Chop the chicken into ½-inch chunks.
2. Brown the chicken in two tablespoons butter using a dutch oven. Transfer it off the hot burner and keep warm.
3. In the same pan, melt the butter. Chop/mince and toss the onion, carrot, celery, and garlic into the pan to sauté until they are tender.
4. Sift and mix in the flour. Slowly mix in the milk, cream, bouillon, and pepper. Wait for it to boil and adjust the temperature setting to low and cook until thickened (2 min.).
5. Add the gnocchi and spinach. Simmer until the spinach is wilted (3-4 min.). Add the chicken. Cover and simmer until heated thoroughly - not boiling - for about ten minutes.

Minestrone Soup

Servings: 8/3 quarts | **Difficulty**: Super Easy | **Time**: 1¼ hours

Nutrition per Serving - 1.5 cups per portion:
- Calories: 191
- Protein: 6 grams
- Fat: 6 grams
- Sat. Fats: 1 gram
- Carbohydrates: 29 grams
- Sugars: 9 grams
- Fiber: 7 grams

Ingredients Needed:
- ☐ Onion (1 large)
- ☐ Olive oil (3 tbsp.)
- ☐ Celery (2 ribs)
- ☐ Cabbage (1 cup)
- ☐ Zucchini (1 medium)
- ☐ Carrots (2 medium)
- ☐ Green pepper (1 medium)
- ☐ Garlic (6 cloves)
- ☐ Water (3.5 cups)
- ☐ Garbanzo beans or Chickpeas (15 oz. can.)
- ☐ Tomato puree (15 oz. can)
- ☐ Diced - undrained tomatoes (2 - 14.5 oz. cans)
- ☐ Tomato sauce (8 oz. can)
- ☐ Salt (1 tsp.)
- ☐ Black pepper (.5 tsp.)
- ☐ Dried parsley flakes (3 tbsp.)
- ☐ Cayenne pepper (.25 tsp.)
- ☐ Dried oregano & basil (2 tsp. each)
- ☐ Pasta shells - small (.5 cup)

Optional Toppings:
- ☐ Fresh leaves of basil
- ☐ Shaved parmesan cheese

Preparation Guidelines:

1. Rinse and drain the beans.
2. Prepare a dutch oven to warm the oil, and sauté the onion for two minutes.
3. Chop and add the celery, carrots, garlic, green pepper, zucchini, and cabbage, Sauté them for three minutes.
4. Stir in the tomatoes (juice too), tomato sauce, water, beans, tomato puree, and seasonings. Wait for the mixture to boil. Reduce the heat setting and cover to cook for another 15 minutes.
5. Fold in the pasta and simmer for 12-15 minutes until tender. Garnish each serving with basil and cheese as desired.

Dinner

Chicken Margherita

Servings: 4 | **Difficulty**: Very Easy | **Time**: 30 min

Nutrition per Serving - 1 cup spaghetti & 1 chicken breast per serving:

- Calories: 431
- Protein: 40 grams
- Fat: 10 grams
- Sat. Fats: 4 grams
- Carbohydrates: 47 grams
- Sugars: 4 grams
- Fiber: 8 grams

Ingredients Needed:

- ☐ Whole-wheat spaghetti (8 oz. uncooked)
- ☐ Chicken breast halves (4 @ 5 oz. each - skinless & boneless)
- ☐ Pepper (.5 tsp.)
- ☐ Bruschetta topping (1 cup - prepared)
- ☐ Shredded Italian cheese blend (.33 cup)
- ☐ Grated parmesan cheese (2 tbsp.)

Preparation Guidelines:

1. Warm the oven broiler. Prepare the spaghetti according to the package instructions and drain in a colander.
2. Use a meat mallet to pound the chicken into a ½-inch thickness. Sprinkle each piece using pepper.
3. Spritz a skillet with cooking oil spray. Cook the chicken using the medium temperature setting for five to six minutes per side.
4. Transfer the meat to an eight-inch square baking pan. Scoop a portion of the bruschetta topping over the chicken and garnish with the cheeses.
5. Broil it about three to four inches from the burner elements (5-6 min.) or until the cheese is golden brown. Serve with the spaghetti.
6. Note: Look for the bruschetta topping in your grocer's deli case or the pasta aisle.

Shrimp Fettuccine Alfredo

Servings: 5 | **Difficulty**: Very Easy | **Time**: 24 min

Nutrition per Serving - 1.5 cup portion:

- Calories: 538
- Protein: 40 grams
- Fat: 16 grams
- Sat. Fats: 7 grams
- Carbohydrates: 56 grams
- Sugars: 9 grams
- Fiber: 3 grams

Ingredients Needed:

- ☐ Uncooked fettuccine (12 oz.)
- ☐ Olive oil - divided (2 tbsp.)
- ☐ Jumbo shrimp (1 lb. - uncooked)
- ☐ Minced garlic (6 cloves)
- ☐ Evaporated milk (12 oz. can)
- ☐ Grated parmesan cheese (.25 cup)
- ☐ Salt (.5 tsp.)
- ☐ Sour cream (.25 cup)
- ☐ Drained crabmeat (.5 lb.)
- ☐ Fresh basil (.25 cup)

Preparation Guidelines:

1. Prepare the fettuccine according to package instructions, and set it to the side for now.
2. Peel and devein the shrimp.
3. Warm one tablespoon of oil in a skillet using the med-high temperature setting.
4. Add the shrimp and simmer until they have turned pink (4 min.). Transfer the batch to a holding container to keep warm for now.
5. Heat the same pan (medium temp) to warm the rest of the oil.
6. Mince and toss in the garlic to sauté for one to two minutes. Mix in the milk and salt and wait for it to boil, continually stirring.
7. Transfer the pan to a cool burner and fold in cheese until melted. Whisk in the sour cream.
8. Combine the mixture with the fettuccine and add the shrimp and crab.
9. Warm and stir in the basil to serve.

Dessert

Raspberry Lemonade Concentrate

Servings: 5 pints of concentrate | **Difficulty**: Medium | **Time**: 40 min

Nutrition per Serving:

- Calories: 319
- Protein: 1 gram
- Fat: 0 grams
- Sat. Fats: 0 grams
- Carbohydrates: 83 grams
- Sugars: 78 grams
- Fiber: 1 gram

Ingredients Needed:

- ☐ Sugar (6 cups)
- ☐ Lemon juice (4 cups)
- ☐ Fresh raspberries (4 lb./14 cups)
- ☐ Chilled ginger ale/tonic water
- ☐ Ice cubes
- ☐ Also Needed: Five heated 1-pint jars

Preparation Guidelines:

1. Rinse and toss the raspberries in a food processor. Place the lid and pulse them until blended. Strain and discard the seeds from the berries, reserving the juice.
2. Pour the juice in a dutch oven, stirring in the sugar. Warm using the med-high temperature setting (190 °Fahrenheit). Do not boil.
3. Transfer the pan from the burner and skim off the accumulated foam.

4. Carefully ladle the hot mixture into the jars - leaving a ¼-inch head-space.
5. Use a clean towel to cleanse the rims and screw on the bands until they're finger-tip tight.
6. Arrange each of the jars into a canner of boiling water. Process the jars for ten minutes. Use tongs and transfer the jars to the countertop to cool.
7. To prepare one serving, mix one pint each of the concentrate and water. Mix thoroughly and serve over ice.

Tiramisu

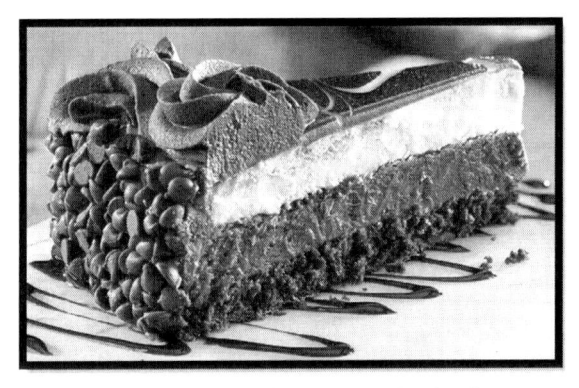

Servings: 12 | **Difficulty**: Simple | **Time**: 25 min

Nutrition per Serving:
- Calories: 321
- Protein: 6 grams
- Fat: 21 grams
- Sat. Fats: 14 grams
- Carbohydrates: 24 grams
- Sugars: 14 grams
- Fiber: 0 grams

Ingredients Needed:

- ☐ Coffee liquor (2 tbsp.)
- ☐ Strong brewed coffee (.5 cup)
- ☐ Sour cream (2 cups)
- ☐ Softened cream cheese (16 oz.)
- ☐ Sugar (2/3 cup)
- ☐ Vanilla extract (.5 tsp.)
- ☐ 2% milk (.25 cup)
- ☐ Ladyfingers - split (2 pkg. @ 3 oz. each)
- ☐ Baking cocoa (1 tbsp.)
- ☐ Also Needed: 11x7-inch baking dish

Preparation Guidelines:

1. Pour and mix the coffee and liqueur.
2. Mix the sugar into the cream cheese in a mixing container. Pour in the milk, vanilla, and sour cream.
3. Layer one of the packages of cookies into the ungreased baking dish, brushing them with half of the coffee mixture. Garnish it using ½ of the cream cheese mixture. Continue the layers and cover using a layer of foil or plastic wrap.
4. Pop the tasty dish into the refrigerator for about eight hours or overnight.
5. Serve with a dusting of cocoa when serving.

Chapter 6:
Chick-fil-A™ Specialties

Breakfast

Chicken Biscuit

Servings: 4 | **Difficulty**: Medium | **Time**: 60 min

Nutrition per Serving:

- Calories: 552
- Protein: 34 grams
- Fat: 20 grams
- Sat. Fats: 10 grams
- Carbohydrates: 58 grams
- Sugars: 11 grams
- Fiber: 2 grams

Ingredients Needed:

The Biscuits:
- ☐ A-P flour (1.25 cups)
- ☐ Salt (.5 tsp.)
- ☐ Baking powder (1 tbsp.)
- ☐ Chilled unsalted butter (.25 cup)
- ☐ Cold buttermilk (.5 cup)
- ☐ Honey (.5 tbsp.)

The Chicken:
- ☐ Dill pickle juice (.33 cup)
- ☐ Milk (2/3 cup)
- ☐ Boneless chicken breast (1 lb.)
- ☐ Eggs (2)
- ☐ Breadcrumbs (.75 cup)

- ☐ Powdered sugar (2 tbsp.)
- ☐ All-Pur. flour (.75 cup)
- ☐ Kosher salt (2 tsp.)
- ☐ Chili powder (.25 tsp.)
- ☐ Black pepper (.5 tsp.)
- ☐ Peanut oil

Preparation Guidelines:

1. Prepare the Biscuits: Preheat the oven at 425° Fahrenheit.
2. Measure and add the salt, flour, and baking powder in a food processor, pulsing to mix.
3. Cube and add the butter to create coarse crumbs, dumping it into a mixing container. Scoop a hole in the center to add the honey and buttermilk. Do not overwork it, stirring with a spatula until just combined.
4. Lightly flour a cutting board. Scoop the dough onto the board, rolling it until it is about one inch thick. Knead the dough to process six times.
5. Gently roll the dough into a rectangular shape until it's about ½-inch thick.
6. Use a three-inch biscuit cutter to make eight biscuits. Scoop the scraps to make another biscuit.
7. Add a layer of parchment baking paper over a baking sheet. Gently brush each biscuit with buttermilk. Set a timer to bake until the tops are golden (15 min.). Transfer to the top of the stovetop and brush with melted butter.
8. Prepare the Chicken: Pound the chicken breasts into a ½-inch thickness and cut in half. Put them into a zipper-type bag with the whisked eggs, milk, and pickle juice. Marinate the chicken in the fridge for about half an hour.
9. Toss the breadcrumbs into the food processor and pulse until they're finely crushed. Toss and whisk the salt, flour, breadcrumbs, sugar, black pepper, and chili powder in a mixing bowl.

10. Dip the breasts of chicken in the mixture and wait for about five minutes before cooking them.
11. Add oil to a cast-iron skillet (½-inch deep) using the medium temperature setting. Cook the chicken in batches if needed for about two to three minutes per side.
12. Slice the freshly made biscuit and serve promptly.

Chicken Egg & Cheese Biscuit

Servings: 5 | **Difficulty**: Medium | **Time**: 45-50 min

Nutrition per Serving - 637-gram serving:
- Calories: 3171.5
- Protein: 46.1 grams
- Fat: 2684 grams
- Sat. Fats: 58.6 grams
- Carbohydrates: 83.7 grams
- Sugars: 10.6 grams
- Fiber: 3.2 grams

Ingredients Needed:
- ☐ Peanut oil for frying (6 cups)

Wet Mixture For The Chicken:
- ☐ Pickle juice (.5 cup)
- ☐ Whole milk (.5 cup)
- ☐ Garlic & onion powder (.5 tsp. each)
- ☐ Chicken thighs (2.5 lb.)
- ☐ Egg (1)

Dry Mixture For The Chicken:
- ☐ A-P flour (3 cups)
- ☐ Baking powder (2 tbsp.)
- ☐ Kosher salt (1 tbsp.)
- ☐ Powdered sugar (.25 cup)
- ☐ Paprika (1 tbsp.)
- ☐ Chili powder (2 tsp.)
- ☐ Refrigerated buttermilk biscuits (6 oz.)

Cheesy Eggs:
- ☐ Cooking oil spray (as needed)
- ☐ Milk (.25 cup)
- ☐ Large eggs (8)
- ☐ Kosher salt (2 tsp.)
- ☐ Cheddar cheese (5 slices)

Preparation Guidelines:

1. Warm the oven according to directions on the package of biscuits.
2. Attach a deep-frying thermometer to the side of a large heavy-bottomed pot or dutch oven. Warm about 2.5 inches of oil using the medium temperature setting (325° Fahrenheit). Cover a baking tray using a few paper towels.
3. Whisk the wet fixings in a medium bowl. Place the chicken into marinade.
4. As the oil heats, whisk the dry ingredients.
5. Reserving the marinade, transfer the chicken to a bowl.
6. Whisk the egg into the marinade. Dip the chicken into the egg mixture, one piece at a time, shaking off excess egg mixture. Dredge chicken pieces in the flour mix, making sure to coat evenly on both sides.
7. Repeat the breading process (egg mixture to flour mixture) one more time, and set chicken aside.
8. Once the oil is heated, cook the chicken for about two to three minutes on each side until well done.
9. As the chicken cooks, prepare the biscuits according to package directions. Place cooked chicken on the prepared baking sheet to drain. Set biscuits aside.
10. Scramble the Eggs: Reset the oven temperature at 350° Fahrenheit. Generously spray a small rimmed baking sheet (9x13) with cooking oil spray. In a medium bowl, reserving the sliced cheddar cheese, whisk the folded egg fixings until pale in color and frothy.
11. Dump the egg mixture into the baking sheet. Cook until the mixture is slightly wobbly, but set in the center, about six to eight minutes, rotating the pan halfway through.

12. Cover the baking tray with a cutting board for about four minutes, or until the egg is set in center, but still tender.
13. With two hands, use kitchen towels to the sandwich baking sheet and cutting board. Flip the "sandwich" over, placing the board on the kitchen counter.
14. Lift the pan and slice the cooked egg crosswise into five even strips. Gently fold each slice in half lengthwise and transfer, using a thin spatula, back onto the baking tray. Top with cheese to bake for two to three minutes, or until the cheese is melted.
15. Split each biscuit in half and top each with chicken, egg, and remaining biscuit top. Serve immediately.

Lunch

Chick-fil-A™ Sandwich

Servings: 4 | **Difficulty**: Fairly Easy | **Time**: 55 min

Nutrition per Serving:

- Calories: 454.6
- Carbohydrates: 44.2 grams
- Protein: 28.6 grams
- Fat: 18.2 grams
- Sat. Fats: 2.9 grams
- Sugars: 7.6 grams
- Fiber: 5.1 grams

Ingredients Needed:

- ☐ Hamburger buns (4 - split)
- ☐ Lettuce (1 head)
- ☐ Dill pickle (20 slices)
- ☐ Sliced tomato (1)
- ☐ Chicken breasts (2)
- ☐ Milk - divided (1.5 cups)
- ☐ Dill pickle juice (1 cup)
- ☐ Egg (1 large)
- ☐ All-purpose flour (.5 cup)
- ☐ Kosher salt and freshly cracked black pepper (as desired)
- ☐ Confectioners' sugar (1 tbsp.)
- ☐ Peanut oil (1 cup)

Preparation Guidelines:

1. Slice the breast of chicken in half - horizontally on a cutting board, trimming away the fat.
2. Whisk the pickle juice and ½ cup milk. Toss in the chicken and marinate it for about 30 minutes. Drain well.
3. Prepare a skillet using the medium-temperature setting to warm the oil.
4. Prepare another container and whisk egg and last cup of milk. Fold in the chicken to coat.
5. In a gallon-sized zipper-type bag, combine the flour, salt, pepper, and confectioners' sugar. Toss in the chicken and shake to cover.
6. Arrange the chicken in the skillet and fry for four to five minutes. (Prepare in batches if needed and drain on paper towels.)
7. Serve the chicken promptly on buns with lettuce, pickles, and tomatoes.

Market Salad

Servings: 4 | **Difficulty**: Easy - Mostly prep | **Time**: 25 min

Nutrition per Serving:
- Calories: 311
- Protein: 30 grams
- Fat: 12 grams
- Sat. Fats: 4 grams
- Carbohydrates: 22 grams
- Sugars: 13 grams
- Fiber: 5 grams

Ingredients Needed:
- ☐ Chicken breast (2)
- ☐ Olive oil (1 tbsp.)
- ☐ Coarse black pepper (⅛ tsp.)
- ☐ Kosher salt (.25 tsp.)
- ☐ Paprika (.25 tsp.)
- ☐ Cayenne pepper (⅛ tsp.)
- ☐ Chopped spring salad mix (16 cups)
- ☐ Blueberries (1 cup)
- ☐ Chopped Granny Smith apple (1)
- ☐ Strawberries (1 cup - halved)
- ☐ Crumbled blue cheese (.5 cup)
- ☐ Granola (1 cup)
- ☐ Roasted walnuts (1 cup)
- ☐ Zesty apple cider vinaigrette (1 cup - below)
    - ☐ Olive oil (.66 cup)
    - ☐ Lime juice (3 tbsp.)
    - ☐ Honey (.25 cup)
    - ☐ Apple cider vinegar (.25 cup)
    - ☐ Black pepper (.5 tsp.)
    - ☐ Garlic powder (.5 tsp.)
    - ☐ Salt (1 tsp.)

Preparation Guidelines:

1. Combine the oil, chicken, cayenne, black pepper, salt, and pepper.
2. Warm a skillet using the medium temperature setting. Cook the chicken for five to eight minutes per side. Cool the chicken and prepare the salad.
3. Prepare the vinaigrette using the listed fixings and shake it thoroughly before using it.
4. Layer the lettuce, cabbage, carrots, strawberries, blueberries, apple, walnuts, granola, and blue cheese. Thinly slice and add the chicken.
5. Spritz with the chilled dressing and serve.

Sweet Carrot Salad

Servings: 8 | **Difficulty**: Super Easy | **Time**: 40 min

Nutrition per Serving:

- Calories: 105
- Protein: 1 gram
- Fat: 2.9 grams
- Sat. Fats: 0.4 grams
- Carbohydrates: 20.6 grams
- Sugars: 15.3 grams
- Fiber: 2.2 grams

Ingredients Needed:

- ☐ Grated carrots (1 lb.)
- ☐ Raisins (.5 cup)
- ☐ Crushed pineapple (1 cup)
- ☐ Lemon juice (1 dash)
- ☐ Honey (1 tbsp.)
- ☐ Mayonnaise (2 tbsp.)

Preparation Guidelines:

1. Chop/mince the carrots, pineapple, and raisins.
2. Mix in the honey, lemon juice, and mayo.
3. Pop it in the fridge for at least half an hour before serving.

Dinner

Chick Nuggets

Servings: 4 | **Difficulty**: Easy | **Time**: 45 min

Nutrition per Serving:

- Calories: 379
- Protein: 33 grams
- Fat: 8 grams
- Sat. Fats: 2 grams
- Carbohydrates: 39 grams
- Sugars: 8 grams
- Fiber: 1 gram

Ingredients Needed:

- ☐ Large eggs (2)
- ☐ Milk (1 cup)
- ☐ Chicken breast (1-inch cubes - 1 lb.)
- ☐ Flour (.75 cup)
- ☐ Breadcrumbs (.75 cup)
- ☐ Powdered sugar (2 tbsp.)
- ☐ White pepper (.5 tsp.)
- ☐ Kosher salt (2 tsp.)
- ☐ Chili powder (.25 tsp.)
- ☐ Peanut oil (3-inches in the skillet)

Preparation Guidelines:

1. Toss the breadcrumbs into a food processor, pulsing until they're fine.
2. Use a zipper-type baggie and add the pieces of chicken, whisked, eggs, and milk.
3. Place the marinated chicken in the fridge for about 15-20 minutes.
4. Pour three inches of oil into a dutch oven and heat using the med-high temperature setting.
5. Measure and whisk the powdered sugar, flour, breadcrumbs, salt, white pepper, and chili powder into a shallow dish.
6. Dip the chicken into the flour mix. Wait a minute and fry in batches (2-3 min.). Transfer them onto a baking tray to serve promptly. Don't use towels to drain because it could soften/steam the nuggets.

Honey Mustard Grilled Chicken

Servings: 4 | **Difficulty**: Easy | **Time**: 35 min

Nutrition per Serving:

- Calories: 265.9
- Protein: 24.7 grams
- Fat: 8.3 grams
- Sat. Fats: 1.6 grams
- Carbohydrates: 22 grams
- Sugars: 17.5 grams
- Fiber: 0.1 grams

Ingredients Needed:

- [ ] Dijon mustard (.33 cup)
- [ ] Honey (.25 cup)
- [ ] Mayonnaise (2 tbsp.)
- [ ] Steak sauce (1 tsp.)
- [ ] Chicken breast halves (4 - no skin or bones)

Preparation Guidelines:

1. Lightly oil the grate and warm the grill using the medium temperature setting.
2. Prepare a shallow dish with the steak sauce, mayo, honey, and mustard. Set aside a portion for basting and rest for the coating sauce.
3. Grill the chicken for about 20 minutes, turning intermittently.
4. Baste using the reserved sauce the last ten minutes of the cooking cycle.

Dessert

Best Lemonade Ever

Servings: 1 | **Difficulty**: Easy | **Time**: 35 min

Nutrition per Serving:

- Calories: 145
- Protein: 0.1 grams
- Fat: 0 grams
- Sat. Fats: 0 grams
- Carbohydrates: 38.2 grams
- Sugars: 36 grams
- Fiber: 0.1 grams

Ingredients Needed:

- ☐ White sugar (1.75 cups)
- ☐ Water (8 cups)
- ☐ Lemon juice (1.5 cups)

Preparation Guidelines:

1. Prepare a saucepan with one cup of water and sugar. Boil until the sugar is dissolved. Cool the mixture until it's room temperature and place it in the fridge (covered) until it's chilled.
2. Clean the lemons and remove the seeds—Juice the lemon with the rest of the water, and chilled syrup.
3. Serve when cold into chilled glasses.

Cookies & Cream Milkshake

Servings: 2 shakes | **Difficulty**: Super Easy | **Time**: 5 min

Nutrition per Serving:
- Calories: 461
- Carbohydrates: 58 grams
- Fat: 22 grams
- Sat. Fats: 11 grams
- Sugars: 43 grams
- Fiber: 2 grams

Ingredients Needed:

- ☐ Oreo cookies (6)
- ☐ Softened - French vanilla ice cream (2.5 cups)
- ☐ Vanilla extract (2 tsp.)

Optional Toppings:
- ☐ Whipped cream (as desired)
- ☐ Maraschino cherries (2)

Preparation Guidelines:

1. Crush the cookies in a blender.
2. Scoop in the ice cream, vanilla extract, and milk.
3. Mix until it's creamy and pour into two chilled mugs.
4. Garnish with a portion of whipped cream and a cherry to your liking. Be sure to add calories (if you are counting).

Peppermint Milkshake

Servings: 3 | **Difficulty**: Super Easy | **Time**: 5-8 min

Nutrition per Serving:

- Calories: 509
- Carbohydrates: 74 grams
- Protein: 7 grams
- Fat: 20 grams
- Sat. Fats: 12 grams
- Sugars: 60 grams
- Fiber: 1 gram

Ingredients Needed:

- ☐ Candy canes (8)
- ☐ Milk (1 cup)
- ☐ Vanilla ice cream (2.5 cups)
- ☐ Peppermint extract (1 tsp.)
- ☐ Semi-sweet chocolate (.25 cup - shaved)

Preparation Guidelines:

1. Prepare the chocolate by shaving it from a semi-sweet baking bar using a veggie peeler or micro-plane grater.
2. Pulse the candy canes in a blender until they are the size of small pebbles.
3. Scoop and add in the ice cream, chocolate, milk, and peppermint extract.
4. Mix it for about ten seconds.
5. Garnish the delicious drink using whipped cream and a cherry.

Chapter 7: Dairy Queen™ Specialties

Brunch

Caramel MooLatte

Servings: 6 | **Difficulty**: Super Easy | **Time**: 20 min

Nutrition per Serving - without the butterscotch topping:

- Calories: 220
- Protein: 3 grams
- Fat: 14 grams
- Sat. Fats: 9 grams
- Carbohydrates: 19 grams
- Sugars: 16 grams
- Fiber: 1 gram

Ingredients Needed:

- ☐ Heavy whipping cream (.5 cup)
- ☐ Confectioner's sugar (1 tbsp.)
- ☐ Dutch-processed cocoa (.25 cup)
- ☐ Vanilla extract - divided (1 tsp.)
- ☐ Half & Half cream (1.5 cups)
- ☐ Hot strong-brew coffee (4 cups)
- ☐ Caramel flavoring syrup (.5 cup)
- ☐ Ice cream topping - Butterscotch-caramel

Preparation Guidelines:

1. Whisk the whipping cream until it begins to thicken. Stir in ½ teaspoon of vanilla and the confectioners' sugar, mixing until stiff peaks form.
2. Prepare a large saucepan using the medium-temperature setting and whisk the cocoa and half-and-half cream until creamy. Warm the mixture until bubbles form around the sides of the pan.
3. Whisk in the caramel syrup, coffee, and rest of the vanilla.
4. Garnish each serving with whipped cream and a drizzle of butterscotch topping.

Turkey BLT

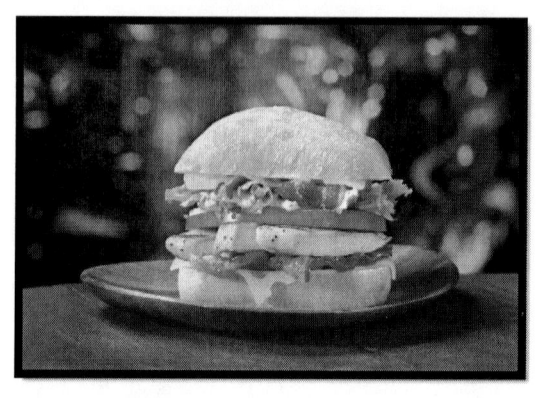

Servings: 4 | **Difficulty**: Super Easy | **Time**: 25 min

Nutrition per Serving:
- Calories: 599
- Protein: 43 grams
- Fat: 25 grams
- Sat. Fats: 7 grams
- Carbohydrates: 46 grams
- Sugars: 11 grams
- Fiber: 2 grams

Ingredients Needed:

- ☐ Boneless & skinless breast of chicken (4 @ 5 oz. each)
- ☐ Salt & Black pepper (.5 tsp. of each)
- ☐ Canola oil (2 tsp.)
- ☐ Tomato slices (4)
- ☐ Processed Swiss cheese (4 slices)
- ☐ Mango chutney (.25 cup)
- ☐ Mayonnaise (3 tbsp.)
- ☐ Split & toasted kaiser rolls (4)
- ☐ Fresh baby spinach (1 cup)
- ☐ Warmed ready-to-serve fully cooked ham (8 slices)

Preparation Guidelines:

1. Flatten the pieces of chicken to about ½-inch thickness. Sprinkle each piece with black pepper and salt.
2. Prepare a large skillet using the medium temperature setting. Cook the chicken in oil for four to five minutes per side until done.
3. Top each chicken breast half with a slice of tomato and cheese. Cover with a lid to cook until the cheese is melted (2-3 min.).
4. Combine the chutney and mayo. Spread the mixture over the roll bottoms. Layer each sandwich with spinach, chicken, and bacon. Replace the tops and serve for a quick and easy meal.

Lunch

DQ Fries

Servings: 6 | **Difficulty**: Super Easy | **Time**: 55 min

Nutrition per Serving - 4 Wedges:

- Calories: 285
- Protein: 10 grams
- Fat: 14 grams
- Sat. Fats: 4 grams
- Carbohydrates: 33 grams
- Sugars: 1 gram
- Fiber: 4 grams

Ingredients Needed:

- ☐ Potatoes (3 large/2.5 lb.)
- ☐ Olive oil (.25 cup)
- ☐ Minced garlic (3 cloves)
- ☐ Dried thyme (.5 tsp.)
- ☐ Seasoned salt (.5 tsp. - divided)
- ☐ Romano-Parmesan cheese blend - divided (.75 cup - grated)
- ☐ Freshly minced parsley (.25 cup)

Preparation Guidelines:

1. Warm the oven setting to reach 425° Fahrenheit. Slice each potato lengthwise into eight wedges and toss them into a large mixing container. Add in the oil, garlic, thyme, and ¼ teaspoon of the seasoned salt, tossing to coat.
2. With a slotted spoon, transfer the potatoes into two greased baking trays. Set oil mixture aside.
3. Roast them for 30 minutes - turning once. Return the potatoes to the oil mixture. Sprinkle with ½ cup of cheese and parsley; toss to coat.
4. Transfer the potatoes onto the baking sheets and roast until brown and tender (10-15 min.).
5. Sprinkle with the rest of the cheese and seasoned salt.

Slow-Cooked Chili Cheese Dog

Servings: 10 | **Difficulty**: Easy | **Time**: 4 hours 20 min

Nutrition per Serving:

- Calories: 419
- Protein: 23 grams
- Fat: 24 grams
- Sat. Fats: 9 grams
- Carbohydrates: 29 grams
- Sugars: 6 grams
- Fiber: 3 grams

Ingredients Needed:

- [ ] Ground beef (1.5 lb.)
- [ ] Yellow onions (2 small - divided)
- [ ] Paprika (.25 tsp.)
- [ ] Ground cinnamon (.5 tsp.)
- [ ] Garlic powder (.25 tsp.)
- [ ] Baking cocoa (1.5 tsp.)
- [ ] Chili powder (.25 tsp.)
- [ ] Worcestershire sauce (2 tbsp.)
- [ ] Tomato sauce (2 - 15 oz. cans)
- [ ] Cider vinegar (1 tbsp.)
- [ ] Hot dogs (10)
- [ ] Split dog buns (10)
- [ ] Shredded cheddar cheese
- [ ] Suggested: 3-quart slow cooker

Preparation Guidelines:

1. Chop the onions.
2. Prepare the ground beef in a large skillet, crumbling the meat until it's no longer pink. Drain it on a layer of paper towels.
3. Toss the beef with one chopped onion, add the next eight ingredients (up to the line).
4. Securely close the lid and set the timer for two hours. Add hot dogs. Continue cooking, covered, on low until heated or about two more hours.
5. Serve on buns; top with shredded cheese and rest of the chopped onion.

Dinner

Flame-Thrower Grill-Burger

Servings: 4 | **Difficulty**: Super Easy Dinner | **Time**: 40 min

Nutrition per Serving:

- Calories: 846
- Protein: 57 grams
- Fat: 50 grams
- Sat. Fats: 21 grams
- Carbohydrates: 40 grams
- Sugars: 4 grams
- Fiber: 5 grams

Ingredients Needed:

- ☐ Ripe avocado (1 medium)
- ☐ Onion (1 small)
- ☐ Tomato (1 medium)
- ☐ Drained jalapeno peppers (4 oz. can - divided)
- ☐ Garlic clove (1)
- ☐ Lime juice (1 tbsp.)
- ☐ Ground beef (2 lb.)
- ☐ Reduced-fat cream cheese (4 oz.)
- ☐ Monterey Jack cheese (1 cup - shredded)
- ☐ Steak seasoning - ex. McCormick's Montreal (1 tbsp.)
- ☐ Split kaiser rolls (4)
- ☐ Bibb lettuce (4 leaves)

Preparation Guidelines:

1. Peel and cube the avocado. Finely chop or mince the onion, tomato, jalapeno, and garlic. Toss it all together with half of the jalapenos, and lime juice; set aside. Shape the mixture into eight patties.
2. In another mixing container, mix the rest of the jalapenos with the cheeses and add it to the center of four patties. Top with the rest of the burger patties - mashing them closed with a spritz of steak seasoning.
3. Grill the burgers using the medium-temperature setting (lid on) for six to seven minutes per side (internal temp of 160° Fahrenheit).
4. Place them on rolls with lettuce and the avocado mixture.

Desserts

DQ™ Banana Split

Servings: 4 | **Difficulty**: Quick & Easy | **Time**: 10 min

Nutrition per Serving:
- Calories: 467
- Protein: 6 grams
- Fat: 15 grams
- Sat. Fats: 9 grams
- Carbohydrates: 84 grams
- Sugars: 63 grams
- Fiber: 5 grams

Ingredients Needed:
- ☐ Bananas (4 medium)
- ☐ Chocolate ice cream (8 scoops)

Ice Cream Toppings (2 tbsp. of each):
- ☐ Pineapple
- ☐ Strawberry
- ☐ Black cherry

Optional Garnishes:
- ☐ Whipped cream
- ☐ Maraschino cherries
- ☐ Chopped pecans

Preparation Guidelines:
1. Slice each banana in half lengthwise.
2. Arrange two banana halves in each of four dessert dishes, and top them with ice cream. Spoon the toppings over the ice cream.
3. Garnish each serving with whipped cream, pecans and a cherry.

DQ™ Round Cake

Servings: 12 | **Difficulty**: Super Easy | **Time**: 50 min

Nutrition per Serving:
- Calories: 374
- Protein: 5 grams
- Fat: 19 grams
- Sat. Fats: 8 grams
- Carbohydrates: 45 grams
- Sugars: 27 grams
- Fiber: 1 gram

Ingredients Needed:

- ☐ Icecream - Birthday cake flavor/your choice (4 cups)
- ☐ Funfetti cake mix (1 regular size box)
- ☐ Thawed - frozen whipped cream (8 oz. carton)
- ☐ Sprinkles
- ☐ Also Needed: 2 Nine-inch round cake pan

Preparation Guidelines:

1. Line the pan with plastic wrap. Spread the ice cream into the pan and freeze it for two hours or until it's firm.
2. Prepare and bake the cake using the two baking pans. Cool it in the pans for about ten minutes before removing to wire racks to thoroughly cool.
3. Using a serrated knife and trim tops of cakes if domed.
4. Place one cake layer on a serving plate. Invert the ice cream onto the cake layer and discard the wrap. Add the last segment of cake and decorate it using the whipped topping.
5. Top it off using sprinkles as desired. Freeze for another two hours longer or until firm.

Oreo Cookie Blizzard

Servings: 1 | **Difficulty**: Super Easy | **Time**: 5 min

Nutrition per Serving:

- Calories: 1157
- Carbohydrates: 144 grams
- Protein: 17 grams
- Fat: 57 grams
- Sat. Fats: 31 grams
- Sugars: 113 grams
- Fiber: 4 grams

Ingredients Needed:

☐ Softened vanilla ice cream (3 cups)
☐ Crushed Oreo cookies (6)

Preparation Guidelines:

1. Transfer the ice cream to the countertop to soften until it starts to melt.
2. Scoop the ice cream into the blender and puree it until it is liquified. Crush and toss in half of the cookies. Bump the speed and pulse once or twice.
3. Serve the Blizzard in a chilled mug with a sprinkle of the other half of the crushed cookies.

S'mores Blizzard Treat

Servings: 4 | **Difficulty**: Easy Peeze | **Time**: 15 min

Nutrition per Serving - ¾ cup portion without syrup:
- Calories: 327
- Protein: 5 grams
- Fat: 12 grams
- Sat. Fats: 7 grams
- Carbohydrates: 50 grams
- Sugars: 39 grams
- Fiber: 1 gram

Ingredients Needed:
- ☐ Large marshmallows (14)
- ☐ 2% milk (.5 cup)
- ☐ Graham crackers (.25 cup)
- ☐ Vanilla ice cream (3 cups)
- ☐ Chocolate syrup (as desired)

Preparation Guidelines:
1. Coarsely crush the crackers.
2. Preheat the oven broiler. Prepare a foil-lined baking tray with a spritz of cooking oil.
3. Place the marshmallows on the tray (single-layered). Broil them about three to four inches from the heat source (15-30 seconds per side) until golden brown. Cool thoroughly.
4. Pour the ice cream and milk into a blender. Cover and process just until combined. Add ten toasted marshmallows, cover, and mix until blended.
5. Divide the milkshake into four chilled glasses topping with crushed crackers and the rest of the toasted marshmallows.
6. Drizzle with chocolate syrup and enjoy it promptly.

Vegan DQ Cupcakes

Servings: 2 | **Difficulty**: Super Easy | **Time**: 5 min

Nutrition per Serving:

- Calories: 536
- Carbohydrates: 74 grams
- Protein: 7 grams
- Fat: 25 grams
- Sugars: 56 grams
- Fiber: 3 grams

Ingredients Needed:

- ☐ Vegan chocolate ice cream (1 cup - divided)
- ☐ Vegan vanilla ice cream (1 cup - divided)
- ☐ Crushed Oreos- (divided (.33 cup)
- ☐ Hot fudge (.33 cup - divided)
- ☐ The Topping: Whipped cream - coconut

Preparation Guidelines:

1. Toss half of the ice cream into two sundae dishes.
2. Decorate it off using hot fudge, crushed cookies, and a scoop of ice cream.
3. Top each of the cakes using coconut whipped cream and sprinkles. Serve and enjoy it promptly.

Chapter 8: KFC™ Specialties

Brunch

Georgia Gold Fried Chicken

Servings: 4 | **Difficulty**: Easy | **Time**: 20 min

Nutrition per Serving:

- Calories: 338
- Carbohydrates: 34 grams
- Protein: 31 grams
- Fat: 9 grams
- Sat. Fats: 0 grams
- Sugars: 0 grams
- Fiber: 1 gram

Ingredients Needed:

- ☐ Dry breadcrumb (1 cup)
- ☐ Dijon mustard - divided (1 tsp. + 2 tbsp.)
- ☐ Honey (3 tbsp.)
- ☐ Butter (2 tbsp.)
- ☐ Skinless-boneless chicken breast halves (4 @ 4 oz. each)

Preparation Guidelines:

1. Flatten the chicken toa ¼-inch thickness using a mallet.
2. In a shallow bowl, combine one teaspoon of mustard and breadcrumbs.
3. In another shallow bowl, whisk the honey and rest of the mustard.
4. Dip the prepared chicken into the honey-mustard mixture, and coat each piece with crumbs.
5. Prepare a skillet with butter using the medium temperature setting. Cook the chicken for four to six minutes per side or until chicken juices run clear when pierced with a fork.
6. Serve with your favorite sides or potatoes or on a biscuit.

KFC™ Biscuits

Servings: 12 | **Difficulty**: Easy | **Time**: 30 min

Nutrition per Serving:

- Calories: 256
- Carbohydrates: 26 grams
- Protein: 4 grams
- Fat: 15 grams
- Sat. Fats: 9 grams
- Fiber: 1 gram
- Sugars: 2 grams

Ingredients Needed:

- ☐ A-P flour (3 cups)
- ☐ Salt (1 tsp.)
- ☐ Sugar (4 tsp.)
- ☐ Baking powder (4 tsp.)
- ☐ Heavy whipping cream (2 cups)

Preparation Guidelines:

1. Warm the oven at 375° Fahrenheit.
2. Whisk the salt, sugar, flour, and baking powder.
3. Fold in the cream, stirring until it's just moistened.
4. Drop 12 of them onto a greased baking sheet.
5. Bake until bottoms are golden brown (17-20 min.). Serve warm.

Lunch

Creamy Coleslaw

Servings: 6 | **Difficulty**: Super Easy | **Time**: 10 min

Nutrition per Serving:
- Calories: 283
- Protein: 1 gram
- Fat: 24 grams
- Sat. Fats: 5 grams
- Carbohydrates: 13 grams
- Sugars: 11 grams
- Fiber: 2 grams

Ingredients Needed:

- ☐ Coleslaw mix (14 oz. pkg.)
- ☐ Mayo (.75 cup)
- ☐ Sour cream (.33 cup)
- ☐ Sugar (.25 cup)
- ☐ Seasoned salt (.75 tsp.)
- ☐ Ground mustard (.5 tsp.)
- ☐ Celery salt (.25 tsp.)

Preparation Guidelines:
1. Toss the coleslaw mix in a large mixing container.
2. Mix and add the rest of the fixings into another container.
3. Combine the fixings and mix well.
4. Pop the slaw in the fridge to chill before serving.

Slow-Cooked Mac & Cheese

Servings: 16 | **Difficulty**: Easy | **Time**: 2 hours 25 min

Nutrition per Serving - ¾ cup portion:
- Calories: 388
- Protein: 17 grams
- Fat: 28 grams
- Sat. Fats: 17 grams
- Carbohydrates: 16 grams
- Sugars: 6 grams
- Fiber: 0 grams

Ingredients Needed:
- ☐ Uncooked elbow macaroni (3 cups)
- ☐ White cheddar shredded cheese (2 cups)
- ☐ Processed cheese - ex. Velveeta (16 oz. pkg. - cubed)
- ☐ Mexican shredded cheese blend (2 cups)
- ☐ Evaporated milk (12 oz. can)
- ☐ Whole milk (1.75 cups)
- ☐ Melted butter (.75 cup)
- ☐ Lightly whisked eggs (3 large)

Preparation Guidelines:

1. Cook the macaroni until it's for al dente (8-10 min.) and drain. Transfer it into a greased five-quart slow cooker. Stir in the rest of the fixings.
2. Cook, covered, using the lowest temperature setting until a thermometer reads at least 160° Fahrenheit or about 2-2.5 hours, stirring once.

Dinner

BBQ Rods

Servings: 4 | **Difficulty**: Super Easy | **Time**: 30 min

Nutrition per Serving:

- Calories: 134
- Protein: 23 grams
- Fat: 3 grams
- Sat. Fats: 1 gram
- Carbohydrates: 1 gram
- Sugars: 1 gram
- Fiber: 0 grams

Ingredients Needed:

- ☐ Plain - reduced-fat yogurt (.75 cup)
- ☐ Lemon juice (1 tbsp.)
- ☐ Olive oil (1 tbsp.)
- ☐ Poultry seasoning (1 tsp.)
- ☐ Salt (.5 tsp.)
- ☐ Oregano (1 tsp. - dried)
- ☐ Onion powder (.25 tsp.)
- ☐ Grated lemon zest (.5 tsp.)
- ☐ Pepper (.25 tsp.)
- ☐ Chicken breasts - skinless and boneless (1 lb. cut into strips)

Preparation Guidelines:

1. Toss each of the fixings in a large mixing container. Toss lightly and pop in the fridge for at least ten minutes or up to eight hours.
2. Trash the marinade and remove the chicken. Thread the chicken onto eight soaked wooden or metal skewers.
3. Arrange the chicken on a greased grill rack. Cover and grill using the medium temperature setting or broil four inches from the heat for five to seven minutes, turning once.

Chili-Lime Fried Chicken

Servings: 24 wings | **Difficulty**: Easy | **Time**: 30 min

Nutrition per Serving:

- Calories: 142
- Protein: 5 grams
- Fat: 8 grams
- Sat. Fats: 1 gram
- Carbohydrates: 12 grams
- Sugars: 9 grams
- Fiber: 0 grams

Ingredients Needed:

- ☐ Whole chicken wings (2.5 lb.)
- ☐ Maple syrup (1 cup)
- ☐ Lime juice (2 tbsp.)
- ☐ Chili sauce (.66 cup)
- ☐ Dijon mustard (2 tbsp.)
- ☐ A-P flour (1 cup)
- ☐ Salt (2 tsp.)
- ☐ Pepper (.25 tsp.)
- ☐ Paprika (2 tsp.)
- ☐ For Frying: Oil

Optional Toppings:
- ☐ Lime wedges
- ☐ Thinly sliced green onions

Preparation Guidelines:

1. Portion the wings into three sections discarding the wing-tip part.
2. Prepare a large saucepan and mix the chili sauce, syrup, lime juice, and mustard.
3. Wait for the mixture to boil, cooking until the liquid is reduced to about one cup.
4. In a shallow dish, whisk the flour, pepper salt, and paprika. Add the wings, tossing to coat.
5. In a deep fryer/ electric skillet, warm the oil to 375° Fahrenheit.
6. Fry the wings in batches for six to eight minutes per side, turning once. Drain them on a layer of paper towels.
7. Dump the wings into a large mixing container and pour in the sauce mixture, tossing to cover.
8. Serve promptly, with sliced green onions, and lime wedges if desired.

KFC™ Original-Style Chicken

Servings: 4 | **Difficulty**: Easy | **Time**: 60 min

Nutrition per Serving:

- Calories: 418
- Protein:n15.4 grams
- Fat Content: 21.7 grams
- Sat. Fats: 2.5 grams
- Carbohydrates: 40.5 grams
- Sugars: 2.6 grams
- Fiber: 2.5 grams

Ingredients Needed:

- ☐ A-P flour (1.5 cups)
- ☐ Chili powder (1 tsp.)
- ☐ Celery salt (.5 tsp.)
- ☐ Paprika (1 tbsp.)
- ☐ Sage (.5 tsp.)
- ☐ Black pepper (1 tsp.)
- ☐ Onion salt (2 tsp.)
- ☐ Garlic powder (.5 tsp.)
- ☐ Ground allspice (.5 tsp.)
- ☐ Dried basil (.5 tsp.)
- ☐ Kosher salt (1 tbsp.)
- ☐ Oregano (.5 tsp.)
- ☐ Marjoram (.5 tsp.)
- ☐ Brown sugar (1 tbsp.)
- ☐ Egg white (1)
- ☐ Whole chicken (2 each - breasts, drumsticks. wings, and thighs)
- ☐ Neutral oil for frying (2 quarts)

Preparation Guidelines:

1. Warm the fryer to 350° Fahrenheit. Thoroughly mix the brown sugar, all of the spices, flour, and salt.
2. Dredge the chicken pieces in the egg white and transfer them to the flour mixture.
3. Wait for 5 minutes for the crust to dry a bit.
4. Fry the chicken in batches. Breasts and wings should take 10-13 minutes. The thighs and legs will probably require more time. Use a thermometer to test the thickest part of the chicken, which will read 165° Fahrenheit when it's done.
5. Drain the chicken on a few paper towels before serving it piping hot.

Sauces

KFC™ Buttermilk Ranch Sauce

Servings: Dressing (1 cup) or Dip (2 cups) | **Difficulty**: Very Easy | **Time**: 10 min

Nutrition per Serving - 2 tbsp. portion:

- Calories: 108
- Protein: 1 gram
- Fat: 27 grams
- Sat. Fats: 7 grams
- Carbohydrates: 1 gram
- Sugars: 1 gram
- Fiber: 0 grams

Ingredients Needed:

- ☐ Dried minced chives (1 tbsp.)
- ☐ Dried oregano (1.5 tsp.)
- ☐ Lemon-pepper seasoning (2 tsp.)
- ☐ Garlic powder (1 tbsp.)
- ☐ Dried parsley flakes (2 tbsp.)
- ☐ Salt (1 tsp.)
- ☐ Dried tarragon (1.5 tsp.)

Additional Ingredients Needed - The Dressing - Each Batch:
- ☐ Mayonnaise (.5 cup.)
- ☐ Buttermilk (.5 cup)

Additional Ingredients Needed - The Dip - Each Batch:
- ☐ Mayonnaise (1 cup)
- ☐ Sour cream (1 cup)

Preparation Guidelines:

1. Whisk the seasonings until thoroughly blended and store in a closed container for up to one year. Shake before using it.
2. Note: You will have four batches for dressing or two for a dip (4 tbsp. of the mix.)
3. Prepare the dressing by whisking the mayo, buttermilk, and one tablespoon of the dry mix. Pop it in the fridge for about one hour before serving time.
4. Prepare the mixture for the dip by combining the sour cream, mayo, and two tablespoons of the dry mixture until blended. Pop it in the refrigerator for about two hours before serving.
5. Enjoy the sauce anytime!

KFC™ Sweet N' Tangy BBQ Sauce

Servings: 1.5 cups | **Difficulty**: Medium | **Time**: 1 hour

Nutrition per Serving - 2 tbsp. portion:

- Calories: 68
- Protein: 0 grams
- Fat: 1 gram
- Sat. Fats: 0 grams
- Carbohydrates: 14 grams
- Sugars: 11 grams
- Fiber: 1 gram

Ingredients Needed:

- ☐ Onion (1 medium-sized)
- ☐ Canola oil (1 tbsp.)
- ☐ Garlic clove (1)
- ☐ Cayenne pepper (.25 tsp.)
- ☐ Chili powder (1-3 tsp.)
- ☐ Coarsely ground pepper (.25 tsp.)
- ☐ Molasses (.33 cup)
- ☐ Ketchup (1 cup)
- ☐ Cider vinegar (2 tbsp.)
- ☐ Hot pepper sauce (.5 tsp.)
- ☐ Spicy brown mustard (2 tbsp.)
- ☐ Worcestershire sauce (2 tbsp.)

Preparation Guidelines:

1. Warm oil in a large saucepan until hot.
2. Chop and sauté the onion until it's tender. Mince and toss in the garlic to sauté for one additional minute. Stir in the cayenne, chili powder, and pepper. Simmer and sauté for one minute.
3. Mix in the molasses, ketchup, Worcestershire sauce, vinegar, mustard, and pepper sauce. Wait for it to boil.
4. Lower the temperature setting to simmer with the lid off for about 30-40 minutes. Cook for another 15 minutes.
5. Use a fine-mesh strainer to strain the sauce over a large mixing container, discarding the seasonings and veggies.
6. Store the sauce in a closed container for up to 30 days in the fridge.

Dessert

Chocolate Chip Cake

Servings: 12 | **Difficulty**: Easy | **Time**: 60 min

Nutrition per Serving:

- Calories: 315
- Protein: 5 grams
- Fat: 11 grams
- Sat. Fats: 2 grams
- Carbohydrates: 52 grams
- Sugars: 34 grams
- Fiber: 1 gram

Ingredients Needed:

- ☐ Sugar (2 cups)
- ☐ Baking powder (1 tsp.)
- ☐ A-P flour (1.75 cups)
- ☐ Baking cocoa (.75 cup)
- ☐ Salt (1 tsp.)
- ☐ Baking soda (2 tsp.)
- ☐ Buttermilk (1 cup)
- ☐ Unchilled eggs (2 large)
- ☐ Strong-brewed coffee (1 cup)
- ☐ Vanilla extract (1 tsp.)
- ☐ Canola oil (.5 cup)
- ☐ Confectioner's sugar (1 tbsp.)
- ☐ Also Needed: 10-inch fluted tube pan

Preparation Guidelines:

1. Warm the oven at 350° Fahrenheit.
2. Lightly grease and flour the pan.
3. Mix the first six dry components (up to the line) in a large mixing container.
4. Whisk and add the eggs, buttermilk, coffee, oil, and vanilla. Beat the mixture using the medium speed for two minutes and dump it into the prepared pan.
5. Bake for 45-50 minutes. Cool the cake for ten minutes before removing it from the pan to a cooling rack. Decorate it using a dusting of the confectioners' sugar and serve.

Chapter 9: Bojangles™ Specialties

Brunch

Bo-Berry Biscuit

Servings: 1 dozen | **Difficulty**: Easy | **Time**: 45 min

Nutrition per Serving:
- Calories: 193
- Protein: 4 grams
- Fat: 5 grams
- Sat. Fats: 3 grams
- Carbohydrates: 35 grams
- Sugars: 18 grams
- Fiber: 1 gram

Ingredients Needed:
- ☐ A-P flour (2 cups)
- ☐ Baking soda (.5 tsp.)
- ☐ Salt (.25 tsp.)
- ☐ Sugar (.5 cup)
- ☐ Baking powder (2 tsp.)
- ☐ Lemon yogurt (1 cup)
- ☐ Unchilled egg (1 large)
- ☐ Melted butter (.25 cup)
- ☐ Grated lemon zest (1 tsp.)
- ☐ Blueberries - Fresh or frozen (1 cup)

The Glaze Ingredients Needed:
- ☐ Grated lemon zest (.5 tsp.)
- ☐ Confectioner's sugar (.5 cup)
- ☐ Lemon juice (1 tbsp.)

Preparation Guidelines:

1. Set the oven temperature at 400° Fahrenheit. Lightly spritz a baking tray with cooking oil spray.
2. Sift the baking soda, flour, sugar, baking powder, and salt.
3. In a separate mixing container, beat the egg, yogurt, melted butter, and lemon zest until blended.
4. Fold in the flour mixture. Gently, mix in the berries.
5. Scoop and add the dough one inch apart onto the prepared pan.
6. Bake them until they're lightly browned (15-18 min.).
7. Combine glaze fixings, stirring until smooth. Drizzle the mixture over the warm biscuits.

Cheddar Bo Biscuit

Servings: 12 | **Difficulty**: Easy | **Time**: 30 min

Nutrition per Serving:

- Calories: 237
- Carbohydrates: 26 grams
- Protein: 7 grams
- Fat: 12 grams
- Sat. Fats: 7 grams
- Sugars: 2 grams
- Fiber: 1 gram

Ingredients Needed:

- A-P flour (3 cups)
- Baking powder (3 tsp.)
- Cream of tartar (.75 tsp.)
- Sugar (1 tbsp.)
- Salt (1 tsp.)
- Cold butter (.5 cup)
- Sharp cheddar shredded cheese (1 cup)
- Minced garlic clove (1)
- Crushed pepper flakes (.25-.5 tsp.)
- 2% milk (1.25 cups)

Preparation Guidelines:

1. Warm the oven at 450° Fahrenheit.
2. Whisk the cream of tartar, flour, salt, baking powder, and sugar.
3. Use a pastry blender to cut in the butter until the mixture is crumbly. Fold in the garlic, cheese, and pepper flakes.
4. Mix in the milk, stirring just until moistened.
5. Drop the dough by heaping ¼ cupfuls about two inches apart onto a greased baking tray.
6. Set the timer and bake the biscuits for 18-20 minutes until golden brown. Serve them piping hot.

Gravy Biscuit

Servings: 2 | **Difficulty**: Easy | **Time**: 15 min

Nutrition per Serving:

- Calories: 337
- Carbohydrates: 14 grams
- Protein: 10 grams
- Fat: 27 grams
- Sat. Fats: 14 grams
- Sugars: 8 grams
- Fiber: 0 grams

Ingredients Needed:

- ☐ Bulk pork sausage (.25 lb.)
- ☐ Butter (2 tbsp.)
- ☐ A-P flour (2-3 tbsp.)
- ☐ Black pepper ⅛ tsp.)
- ☐ Salt (.25 tsp.)
- ☐ Whole milk (1.25-1.33 cups)
- ☐ Warm biscuits

Preparation Guidelines:

1. Cook sausage in a skillet using the medium temperature setting until no longer pink. Drain the grease and add the butter, heating until melted.
2. Stir in the flour, pepper, and salt. Simmer, gradually stirring and adding the milk. Once it's boiling, stir until thickened (2 min.).
3. Serve with tasty Bo biscuits.

Plain Biscuit Specialty

Servings: 10 | **Difficulty**: Easy | **Time**: 30 min

Nutrition per Serving:

- Calories: 142
- Protein: 3 grams
- Fat: 5 grams
- Sat. Fats: 1 gram
- Carbohydrates: 20 grams
- Sugars: 1 gram
- Fiber: 1 gram

Ingredients Needed:

- ☐ Baking soda (.5 tsp.)
- ☐ A-P flour (2 cups)
- ☐ Salt (.5 tsp.)
- ☐ Baking powder (2 tsp.)
- ☐ Shortening (.25 cup)
- ☐ Buttermilk (.75 cup)

Preparation Guidelines:

1. Warm the oven at 450° Fahrenheit.
2. Whisk in the flour, salt, baking powder, and soda.
3. Cut in shortening until it's coarsely crumbled. Stir in buttermilk and gently knead the dough.
4. Roll out to ½-inch thickness. Cut the biscuits out using a glass or biscuit cutter and arrange them onto a lightly greased baking tray.
5. Bake until golden brown (10-15 min.).

Stuffed Potato Pancakes

Servings: 8 | **Difficulty**: Easy | **Time**: 25 min

Nutrition per Serving - For two pancakes:

- Calories: 491
- Protein: 12 grams
- Fat Content: 34 grams
- Sat. Fats: 12 grams
- Carbohydrates: 35 grams
- Sugars: 3 grams
- Fibers: 2 grams

Ingredients Needed:

- ☐ Mashed potatoes (2 cups with additional milk & butter)
- ☐ Shredded cheddar cheese (.66 cup)
- ☐ Flour - All-purpose (.33 cup)
- ☐ Large egg (1)
- ☐ Minced chives (1 tbsp.)
- ☐ Black pepper & salt (.5 tsp. each)
- ☐ Seasoned breadcrumbs (.66 cup)
- ☐ Cayenne pepper (.5 tsp.)
- ☐ Onion powder (1 tsp.)
- ☐ Garlic powder (1 tsp.)
- ☐ Unchilled cream cheese (.33 cup)
- ☐ Oil for deep-fat frying needs

Preparation Guidelines:

1. Combine the chives, whisked egg, flour, cheddar cheese, mashed potatoes, pepper, and salt in a large mixing container.
2. In a shallow container, combine the breadcrumbs, onion powder, garlic powder, and cayenne.
3. Shape two teaspoons of the cream cheese into a ball.
4. Wrap ¼ cup of the potato mixture around the cheese ball to cover it completely. Drop into a crumb mixture. Gently coat and shape into a ½-inch thick patty. Repeat with the rest of the cream cheese and potato mixture until you have eight cakes.
5. Use a deep-fat fryer or electric skillet to warm the oil to reach 375° Fahrenheit.
6. Fry the stuffed pancakes, a few at a time until browned (about one to two minutes per side).
7. Place them briefly on a layer of paper towels before serving.

Lunch

Dirty Rice

Servings: 4 | **Difficulty**: Very Easy | **Time**: 30 min

Nutrition per Serving:
- Calories: 461
- Protein: 35 grams
- Fat: 12 grams
- Sat. Fats: 3 grams
- Carbohydrates: 52 grams
- Sugars: 6 grams
- Fiber: 4 grams

Ingredients Needed:
- ☐ Hot - lean turkey breakfast sausage (16 oz. pkg.)
- ☐ Large onion (1)
- ☐ Green pepper (1 medium)
- ☐ Chicken broth - low-sodium (14.5 oz can)
- ☐ Diced tomatoes with garlic & onion (14.5 oz. can)
- ☐ Cajun seasoning (3 tsp.)
- ☐ Pepper (.25 tsp.)
- ☐ Boil-in-bag white rice (2 bags)
- ☐ Optional: Louisiana-style hot sauce

Preparation Guidelines:
1. Prepare a large skillet using the med-high temperature setting. Chop and add the sausage, onion, and peppers to sauté for five to seven minutes.
2. Pour in the rice from the bags, broth, tomatoes, pepper, and Cajun seasoning.
3. Place a lid on the pot, lower the temperature setting, and simmer until the liquid is absorbed (8-10 min.). If desired, serve with hot sauce.

Jambalaya Bowl - Slow-Cooked

Servings: 11 | **Difficulty**: Easy | **Time**: 35 minutes (+) 4.5 hours cook time

Nutrition per Serving:

- Calories: 230
- Carbohydrates: 9 grams
- Protein: 20 grams
- Fat: 13 grams
- Sat. Fats: 5 grams
- Sugars: 5 grams
- Fiber: 2 grams

Ingredients Needed:

- ☐ Chicken/beef broth (14.5 oz. can)
- ☐ Undrained diced tomatoes (14.5 oz. can)
- ☐ Tomato paste (6 oz. can)
- ☐ Celery (3 ribs)
- ☐ Medium onion (1)
- ☐ Green peppers (2 medium)
- ☐ Garlic (5 cloves)
- ☐ Dried basil (2 tsp.)
- ☐ Dried parsley flakes (3 tsp.)
- ☐ Dried oregano (1.5 tsp.)
- ☐ Cayenne pepper (.5 tsp.)
- ☐ Salt (1.25 tsp.)
- ☐ Hot pepper sauce (.5 tsp.)
- ☐ Chicken breasts (1-inch cubes/1 lb.)
- ☐ Smoked sausage (halved - .25-inch cubes/1 lb)
- ☐ Uncooked medium shrimp (.5 lb.)
- ☐ Hot prepared rice
- ☐ Also Needed: 5-quart slow cooker

Preparation Guidelines:

1. Peel and devein the shrimp.
2. Prepare the cooker by adding the tomatoes, tomato paste, and broth.
3. Chop and stir in the celery, green peppers, onion, garlic, seasonings, and pepper sauce. Fold in the chicken and sausage.
4. Cover and cook using the low-temperature setting for four to six hours.
5. Stir in the shrimp. Place a lid on the cooker and simmer for 15-30 minutes longer until shrimp turns pink.
6. Serve with a portion of rice.

Dinner

"Bojangler" On-the-Go

Servings: 4 sandwiches | **Difficulty**: Quick & Easy | **Time**: 30 min

Nutrition per Serving:

- Calories: 277
- Protein: 31 grams
- Fat: 4 grams
- Sat. Fats: 1 gram
- Carbohydrates: 29 grams
- Fiber: 4 grams

Ingredients Needed:

- ☐ Breadcrumbs (.5 cup)
- ☐ Cayenne pepper (.5 tsp.)
- ☐ Garlic powder (.5 tsp.)
- ☐ Dried parsley flakes (.5 tsp.)
- ☐ Cod fillets (4 @ 6 oz. each)
- ☐ Whole-wheat burger buns - split (4 whole)
- ☐ Plain yogurt (.25 cup)
- ☐ Lemon juice (2 tsp.)
- ☐ Fat-free mayo (.25 cup)
- ☐ Sweet pickle relish (2 tsp.)
- ☐ Dried minced onion (.25 tsp.)
- ☐ Tomato slices (4)
- ☐ Lettuce leaves (4)
- ☐ Sweet onion (4 slices)

Preparation Guidelines:

1. Lightly oil a grill rack and preheat the grill using the medium temperature setting. You can also broil it in the oven at about four to five inches from the heating element,
2. First, prepare a shallow bowl with the breadcrumbs, cayenne, parsley, and garlic powder. Dip the fish into the mixture.
3. Arrange the fish on the grill with the *lid on* for four to five minutes per side until the fish flakes easily.
4. Grill the buns using the medium temperature setting until toasted as desired (1 min.).
5. In the meantime, whisk the mayo, yogurt, relish, minced onion, and lemon juice. Use a butter knife to spread the mixture over the base of the buns.
6. Top the sandwich off with the prepared fish, lettuce, onion, and tomato, adding the top bun to serve.

Homestyle Tenders

Servings: 4 | **Difficulty**: Easy | **Time**: 25 min

Nutrition per Serving - 3 oz. portion:
- Calories: 194
- Carbohydrates: 14 grams
- Protein: 31 grams
- Fat: 2 grams
- Sat. Fats: 0 grams
- Sugars: 1 gram
- Fiber: 1 gram

Ingredients Needed:
- ☐ Egg (1 large) or Egg substitute (.33 cup)
- ☐ Prepared mustard (1 tbsp.)
- ☐ Breadcrumbs (.75 cup)
- ☐ Minced garlic (1 clove)
- ☐ Black pepper (.25 tsp.)
- ☐ Paprika (1 tsp.)
- ☐ Dried basil (2 tsp.)
- ☐ Salt (.5 tsp.)
- ☐ Chicken tenderloins (1 lb.)

Preparation Guidelines:

1. Set the oven temperature at 400° Fahrenheit. Prepare a baking tray with a spritz of cooking oil spray.
2. Use a shallow bowl to whisk the egg substitute, garlic, and mustard.
3. In another shallow bowl, toss the breadcrumbs with the seasonings.
4. Dredge the chicken into the egg and the crumb mixture.
5. Arrange each piece on the baking tray and bake until they are as you like them - crispy and browned (10-15 min.).

Dessert

Legendary Bo Sweet Iced Tea Concentrate

Servings: 20/5 cups of concentrate | **Difficulty**: Easy | **Time**: 30 min

Nutrition per Serving - for ¼ cup of the concentrate:

- Calories: 165
- Protein: 0 grams
- Fat: 0 grams
- Sat. Fats: 0 grams
- Carbohydrates: 43 grams
- Sugars: 40 grams
- Fiber: 0 grams

Ingredients Needed:

- ☐ Lemons (2 medium)
- ☐ Sugar (4 cups)
- ☐ Water (4 cups)
- ☐ English breakfast tea (1.5 cups) or black tea bags (20)
- ☐ Lemon juice (.33 cup)

For Each Serving:
- ☐ Ice cubes
- ☐ Water (1 cup - cold)

Preparation Guidelines:

1. Remove the peels from lemons, saving the fruit for another use.
2. Heat the sugar and water in a large saucepan using the medium-temperature setting until it's boiling.
3. Lower the temperature and simmer, uncovered, until sugar is dissolved (3-5 min.), stirring occasionally.
4. Transfer the pan to a cool burner and add the peels of the lemon and tea leaves. Place a lid on the pan and allow the tea to steep for about 15 minutes.
5. Strain the tea through a mesh strainer, discarding the lemon peels and tea leaves. Cool the tea until it's room temperature and stir in the lemon juice.
6. Pour the tea into a closed top beverage container. Enjoy the drink from the fridge for up to two weeks.
7. Prep the tea in a tall chilled glass, by combining the water with the concentrate (¼ cup) and ice.

Sweet Potato Pie

Servings: 8 | **Difficulty**: Easy | **Time**: 1 ¼ hours

Nutrition per Serving:
- Calories: 513
- Protein: 5 grams
- Fat: 21 grams
- Sat. Fats: 12 grams
- Carbohydrates: 77 grams
- Sugars: 54 grams
- Fiber: 1 gram

Ingredients Needed:
- ☐ A-P flour (3 tbsp.)
- ☐ Sugar (1- 2/3 cups)
- ☐ Salt (1 pinch)
- ☐ Ground nutmeg (.25 tsp.)
- ☐ Mashed sweet potatoes (1 cup)
- ☐ Light corn syrup (.25 cup)
- ☐ Large eggs (2)
- ☐ Evaporated milk (.75 cup)
- ☐ Unchilled butter (.5 cup)
- ☐ Unbaked pastry shell (9-inch)

Preparation Guidelines:

1. Warm the oven to reach 350° Fahrenheit.
2. Sift or whisk the sugar, salt, flour, and nutmeg.
3. In a large mixing container, combine the eggs, butter, potatoes, corn syrup, and sugar mixture. Slowly mix in the milk and dump it into the pastry shell.
4. Bake for 55 minutes to one hour. Transfer it to a wire rack to cool for one hour. Pop it in the fridge for a minimum of three hours before serving.

Chapter 10: Starbucks™

Breakfast

Berry Trio Yogurt

Servings: 8 | **Difficulty**: Easy | **Time**: 20 min

Nutrition per Serving:

- Calories: 304
- Carbohydrates: 54 grams
- Protein: 17 grams
- Fat: 4 grams
- Sat. Fats: 0 grams
- Sugars: 27 grams
- Fiber: 9 grams

Ingredients Needed:

- ☐ Unsweetened raspberries (frozen - 6.5 cups)
- ☐ Packed brown sugar (.25 cup)
- ☐ Cornstarch (2 tbsp.)
- ☐ Orange juice (.25 cup)
- ☐ Fresh blueberries (2 cups)
- ☐ Orange zest (.5 tsp.)
- ☐ Granola - no raisins (2 cups)
- ☐ Fresh blackberries (2 cups)
- ☐ Vanilla greek yogurt (4 cups)
- ☐ Optional: Brown sugar

Preparation Guidelines:

1. Rinse and toss the raspberries and brown sugar in a blender. Close the lid and process until pureed. Press the mixture through a sieve and discard the seeds.
2. Grate the orange zest and combine it with the orange juice, raspberry puree, and cornstarch in a saucepan. Prepare it using the medium temperature setting until thickened and bubbly. Adjust the temp to low, and cook - stirring two minutes longer. Transfer to a cool burner for a few minutes to cool down.
3. Prepare eight parfait glasses, layering half of the raspberry sauce, berries, granola, and yogurt. Repeat the layers and sprinkle with additional brown sugar if desired. Serve promptly.

Chocolate Chunk Muffins

Servings: 12 | **Difficulty**: Easy | **Time**: 40 min

Nutrition per Serving:

- Calories: 308
- Carbohydrates: 45 grams
- Protein: 5 grams
- Fat: 13 grams
- Sat. Fats: 8 grams
- Sugars: 28 grams
- Fiber: 1 gram

Ingredients Needed:

- ☐ Softened butter (.5 cup)
- ☐ Sugar (1 cup)
- ☐ Unchilled eggs (2 large)
- ☐ Plain yogurt (1 cup)
- ☐ Vanilla extract (1 tsp.)
- ☐ Baking powder (.5 tsp.)
- ☐ All-Pur. flour (2 cups)
- ☐ Baking soda (1 tsp.)
- ☐ Salt (.5 tsp.)
- ☐ Semi-sweet chocolate chips (.75 cup)

The Topping:
- ☐ Cinnamon (1 tsp.)
- ☐ Brown sugar (2 tbsp.)
- ☐ Semi-sweet chocolate chips (.25 cup)
- ☐ Optional: Chopped walnuts (2 tbsp.)

Preparation Guidelines:

1. Prepare a mixing container to cream the butter and sugar until it's fluffy.
2. Break in the eggs, stirring thoroughly after adding each one.
3. Whisk in the vanilla and yogurt. Whisk the flour, baking soda, baking powder, and salt, adding it to the creamed mixture - just until moistened.
4. Mix in the chocolate chips. Pour the batter into 12 paper-lined muffin cups (2/3 full.
5. Combine the topping goodies and sprinkle it over the batter.
6. Bake at 350° Fahrenheit for 25-30 minutes. Cool for about five minutes before removing from the pan to a wire rack to cool for storage as desired. Serve warm.

Egg Salad Sandwich

Servings: 3 cups | **Difficulty**: Quick & Easy | **Time**: 10 min

Nutrition per Serving:

- Calories: 228
- Carbohydrates: 6 grams
- Protein: 9 grams
- Fat: 19 grams
- Sat. Fats: 6 grams
- Sugars: 4 grams
- Fiber: 0 grams

Ingredients Needed:

- ☐ Hard-boiled eggs (8 large)
- ☐ Unchilled cream cheese (3 oz.)
- ☐ Mayonnaise (.25 cup)
- ☐ Pepper (1/8 tsp.)
- ☐ Salt (.5 tsp.)
- ☐ Red/green sweet pepper (.25 cup)
- ☐ Celery (.25 cup)
- ☐ Fresh parsley (2 tbsp.)
- ☐ Sweet pickle relish (.25 cup)

Preparation Guidelines:

1. Combine the mayo, salt, pepper, and cream cheese until it's creamy smooth.
2. Finely chop and add the celery, green pepper, parsley, and relish.
3. Chop and fold in the eggs.
4. Cover and chill before serving.

Sausage - Cheddar & Egg Breakfast Sandwich

Servings: 8 | **Difficulty**: Very Easy | **Time**: 40 min

Nutrition per Serving:

- Calories: 741
- Carbohydrates: 31 grams
- Protein: 24 grams
- Fat: 58 grams
- Sat. Fats: 22 grams
- Sugars: 8 grams
- Fiber: 3 grams

Ingredients Needed:

- ☐ Crumbled blue cheese (4 oz./1 cup)
- ☐ Jalapeno (1 pepper - seeded)

Dry Seasonings - 1 tsp. of each:
- ☐ Parsley flakes
- ☐ Oregano
- ☐ Dried basil
- ☐ Bulk Italian sausage (1 lb.)
- ☐ Eggs (8 large)
- ☐ 2% milk (3 tbsp.)
- ☐ Black pepper & salt (1/8 tsp. each)
- ☐ Butter (3 tbsp.)
- ☐ Mayo (.5 cup)
- ☐ Split croissants (8)
- ☐ Slices of tomato (8)
- ☐ Ripe avocado (1 medium)

Preparation Guidelines:

1. Mince the jalapeno and mix with the cheese and herbs. Crumble in and mix with the sausage. Shape the mixture into eight patties.
2. Prepare the patties in a skillet using the medium temperature setting for four to five minutes per side. Keep them warm.
3. Whisk the milk, eggs, pepper, and salt. Prepare another skillet and melt half of the butter using the med-high temperature setting. Add half of the egg to the pan and swirl in the pan until fully cooked. Cover with a lid on the pot for one to two minutes.
4. Set the first eggs aside and repeat the process using the rest of the butter.
5. Slice the first batch into wedges.
6. Peel and slice the avocado.
7. Prepare the croissants with a portion of mayo, patty, eggs, avocado, and tomato. Replace the top and serve!

Starbucks™ Pumpkin Bread

Servings: 10 | **Difficulty**: Easy | **Time**: 1 hour 10 min

Nutrition per Serving:

- Calories: 274
- Protein: 3 grams
- Fat Content: 13 grams
- Sat. Fats: 9 grams
- Carbohydrates: 36 grams
- Sugars: 20 grams
- Fiber: 1 gram

Ingredients Needed:

- ☐ All-purpose flour (1.5 cups)
- ☐ Cardamom (.25 tsp.)
- ☐ Nutmeg (.5 tsp.)
- ☐ Allspice (.25 tsp.)
- ☐ Cinnamon (.5 tsp.)
- ☐ Clove (.25 tsp.)
- ☐ Sugar (1 cup)
- ☐ Salt (.75 tsp.)
- ☐ Baking soda (1 tsp.)
  Note: If you use pumpkin spice, use a scant two tsp. of the spices mentioned
- ☐ Pumpkin puree (1 cup)
- ☐ Eggs (2)
- ☐ Vegetable oil (.5 cup)
- ☐ Roasted & salted pumpkin seeds (.33 cup)
- ☐ Vanilla (.5 tsp.)

Preparation Guidelines:

1. Warm the oven in advance to reach 350° Fahrenheit. Lightly spritz a 9x5x3-inch baking dish using a cooking oil spray.
2. Sift or whisk all of the dry fixings in a large mixing container (spices, salt, baking soda, sugar, and flour). Set aside.
3. Whisk the eggs, oil, puree, and vanilla. Add to the dry ones and mix well until it's lump-free.
4. Pour the mixture into the prepared pan with a sprinkling of pumpkin seeds on its top.
5. Bake for 50-60 minutes until done. Test for doneness using a cake tester or toothpick.
6. Cool for about five minutes before removing it from the pan and placing it on a cooling rack. It's best to cut the bread when it's cooled.
7. *Special Note*: Don't use olive or peanut oil

Lunch or Dinner

Roasted Tomato & Mozzarella Panini

Servings: 4 | **Difficulty**: Easy | **Time**: 10 min

Nutrition per Serving:
- Calories: 435
- Carbohydrates: 31 grams
- Protein: 15 grams
- Fat: 29 grams
- Sat. Fats: 14 grams
- Sugars: 14 grams
- Fiber: 3 grams

Ingredients Needed:
- ☐ Walnut-raisin bread (8 slices)
- ☐ Prepared pesto (3-4 tbsp.)
- ☐ Mozzarella-provolone cheese blend (8 slices)
- ☐ Tomato slices (8)
- ☐ Unchilled butter (.25 cup)

Preparation Guidelines:

1. Spread four slices of bread with the pesto. Layer with the cheese and tomato, adding the bread tops. Butter the outsides of each of the four sandwiches.
2. Use the medium temperature setting to warm a large skillet. Toast the sandwiches for two to three minutes per side or until the cheese is melted and it is nicely browned as desired.

Turkey & Havarti Sandwich

Servings: 8 | **Difficulty**: Super Easy | **Time**: 15 min

Nutrition per Serving:

- Calories: 302
- Carbohydrates: 45 grams
- Protein: 16 grams
- Fat: 7 grams
- Sat. Fats: 2 grams
- Sugars: 9 grams
- Fiber: 2cgrams

Ingredients Needed:

- ☐ Mango chutney (.33 cup)
- ☐ Mayo (2 tbsp. red-fat)
- ☐ Unsalted chopped peanuts (2 tbsp.)
- ☐ Cayenne pepper (1 dash)
- ☐ French bread - halved lengthwise (1 lb. loaf)
- ☐ Lettuce (6 leaves
- ☐ Deli turkey (.75 lb. thinly sliced)
- ☐ Havarti cheese - thinly sliced (2 oz.)
- ☐ Red Delicious apple (1 medium)

Preparation Guidelines:
1. Peel and thinly slice the apple into rings.
2. Mix the mayo, chutney, cayenne, and peanuts, spreading it over the cut side of the bread's bottom.
3. Layer using the lettuce, turkey, cheese, and apple rings. Place the bun top and slice evenly into eight slices.

Dessert

Blueberry Scone

Servings: 16 | **Difficulty**: Super Easy | **Time**: 35 min

Nutrition per Serving:

- Calories: 220
- Carbohydrates: 31 grams
- Protein: 5 grams
- Fat: 9 grams
- Sat. Fats: 5 grams
- Sugars: 7 grams
- Fiber: 1 gram

Ingredients Needed:

- ☐ Flour (4 cups-all-purpose)
- ☐ Sugar (6 tbsp.)
- ☐ Baking powder (4.5 tsp.)
- ☐ Salt (.5 tsp.)
- ☐ Cold butter (.5 cup + 2 tbsp.)
- ☐ Whole milk - divided (.75 cup + 2 tbsp.)
- ☐ Unchilled eggs (2 large)
- ☐ Frozen or fresh blueberries (1.5 cups)

Preparation Guidelines:

1. Warm the oven at 375° Fahrenheit.
2. Whisk the flour, sugar, baking powder, and salt in a mixing container, and cut in the butter until it is coarse crumbs.
3. In a separate mixing container, whisk the eggs and ¾ cup of milk. Stir them into the dry fixings until it's just until moistened. Scoop the dough onto a lightly floured surface and gently mix in the blueberries.
4. Divide the dough in half. Pat each portion into an eight-inch circle, cutting each one into eight wedges. Arrange them on greased baking trays. Brush with remaining milk.
5. Set a timer and bake them until the tops are golden brown (15-20 min.).
6. Enjoy them right out of the oven.

Cranberry Bliss Bar

Servings: 30 | **Difficulty**: Easy-Medium | **Time**: 55 min

Nutrition per Serving:

- Calories: 236
- Protein: 2 grams
- Fat: 11 grams
- Sat. Fats: 6 grams
- Carbohydrates: 32 grams
- Sugars: 24 grams
- Fiber: 0 grams

Ingredients Needed:

- ☐ Cubed butter (.75 cup)
- ☐ Unchilled large eggs (2)
- ☐ Light brown sugar - tightly packed (1.5 cups)
- ☐ Vanilla extract (.75 tsp.)
- ☐ A-P flour (2.25 cups)
- ☐ Salt (.25 tsp.)
- ☐ Cinnamon (.125 tsp.)
- ☐ Baking powder (1.5 tsp.)
- ☐ Dried cranberries (.5 cup)
- ☐ Coarsely chopped white baking chocolate (6 oz.)

The Frosting:
- ☐ Unchilled cream cheese (8 oz. pkg.)
- ☐ Confectioner's sugar (1 cup)
- ☐ Melted white baking chocolate (6 oz.)
- ☐ Chopped dried cranberries (.5 cup)
- ☐ Optional: Grated orange zest (1 tbsp.)
- ☐ Also Needed: 13x9-inch pan

Preparation Guidelines:

1. Set the oven to reach 350° Fahrenheit.
2. Melt the butter in a microwave-safe container, mixing in the brown sugar. Cool the mixture slightly.
3. Mix in one egg at a time, and stir in the vanilla.
4. In another container, whisk the baking powder, salt, flour, and cinnamon. Shake it into the butter mixture and fold in the cranberries and chopped chocolate. Spread the thick batter into a greased baking pan.
5. Bake it until it's nicely browned (18 to 21 min.), but don't overbake. Cool it on a wire rack.
6. Prepare the frosting. Mix the confectioners' sugar, cream cheese, and orange zest until smooth. Gradually mix in ½ of the melted white chocolate, spreading it over the blondies.
7. Sprinkle it using the cranberries and drizzle with the remaining melted chocolate.
8. Use a sharp knife to slice it into triangles. Place them in a container in the fridge.

Cranberry Orange Scone

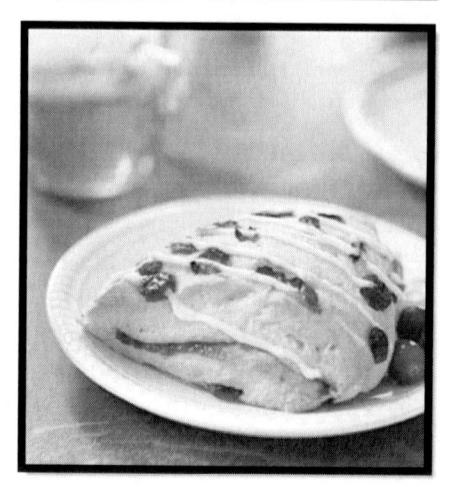

Servings: 10 scones | **Difficulty**: Medium | **Time**: 35 min

Nutrition per Serving:

- Calories: 331
- Carbohydrates: 43 grams
- Protein: 4 grams
- Fat: 17 grams
- Sat. Fats: 10 grams
- Sugars: 22 grams
- Fiber: 1 gram

Ingredients Needed:

- ☐ A-P flour (2 cups)
- ☐ Sugar (10 tsp. divided)
- ☐ Orange zest (1 tbsp.)
- ☐ Salt (.5 tsp.)
- ☐ Baking powder (2 tsp.)
- ☐ Baking soda (.25 tsp.)
- ☐ Dried cranberries (1 cup)
- ☐ Cold butter (.33 cup)
- ☐ Orange juice (.25 cup)
- ☐ Half & Half cream (.25 cup)

- ☐ Unchilled egg (1 large)
- ☐ 2% milk (1 tbsp.)

Optional: The Glaze:
- ☐ Confectioner's sugar (.5 cup)
- ☐ Orange juice (1 tbsp.)

The Orange Butter:
- ☐ Softened butter (.5 cup)
- ☐ Orange marmalade (2-3 tbsp.)

Preparation Guidelines:

1. Combine the flour, grated orange zest, baking powder, seven teaspoons sugar, salt, and baking soda.
2. Mix in the butter using a pastry blender until the mixture is crumbly and set aside.
3. Toss the cranberries with the egg, cream, and orange juice. Add it to the flour mixture and stir into a soft dough.
4. Scoop the dough onto a floured surface to gently knead six to eight times, working it into an eight-inch circle. Slice it into ten wedges.
5. Separate the wedges and arrange them on a greased baking tray. Brush with milk and sprinkle with the rest of the sugar.
6. Bake at 400° Fahrenheit until lightly browned (12-15 min.). Transfer it onto a wire rack.
7. Combine the glaze fixings and drizzle it over the scones.
8. Combine the orange butter ingredients and serve with the warm scones.

Iced Lemon Pound Cake

Servings: 2 mini-loaves/6 slices in each pan | **Difficulty**: Easy | **Time**: 55 min

Nutrition per Serving:

- Calories: 262
- Carbohydrates: 39 grams
- Protein: 3 grams
- Fat: 10 grams
- Sat. Fats: 6 grams
- Sugars: 25 grams
- Fiber: 1 gram

Ingredients Needed:

- ☐ Unchilled butter (.5 cup)
- ☐ Sugar (1 cup)
- ☐ Unchilled eggs (2 large)
- ☐ Vanilla extract (1 tsp.)
- ☐ Grated lemon zest (1 tsp.)
- ☐ Lemon extract (.5 tsp.)
- ☐ Salt (.5 tsp.)
- ☐ A-P flour (1.75 cups)
- ☐ Baking soda (.25 tsp.)
- ☐ Sour cream (.5 cup)

The Icing:
- ☐ Grated lemon zest (.5 tsp.)
- ☐ Confectioner's sugar (.75 cup)
- ☐ Lemon juice (1 tbsp.)
- ☐ Also Needed: Two 5-3/4x3x2-inch loaf pans

Preparation Guidelines:

1. Set the oven temperature at 350° Fahrenheit. Grease and flour the pans.
2. Cream the sugar and butter until it's fluffy. Whisk in one egg at a time, mixing thoroughly after each addition. Mix in the lemon zest and extracts.
3. In another mixing container, whisk the flour, salt, and baking soda, adding it to the creamed mixture alternately with sour cream, mixing fully after each egg is added.
4. Transfer the mixture to the prepared pans. Bake the cake until done (35-40 min.) Test using a toothpick inserted in the center; if it comes out clean - it's done.
5. Cool in pans for ten minutes before removing to wire racks to cool completely.
6. Mix the icing fixings and spoon it over the loaves.

Beverages

Chai Latte

Servings: 6 | **Difficulty**: Easy | **Time**: 25 min

Nutrition per Serving:

- Calories: 102
- Carbohydrates: 17 grams
- Protein: 3 grams
- Fat: 3 grams
- Sat. Fats: 2 grams
- Sugars: 16 grams
- Fiber: 0 grams

Ingredients Needed:

- ☐ Cardamom pods (6)
- ☐ Whole peppercorns (.5 tsp.)
- ☐ Water (5 cups)
- ☐ Honey (.25 cup)
- ☐ Cinnamon sticks (3-inches/2)
- ☐ Whole cloves (8)
- ☐ Freshly minced ginger root (1 tbsp.)
- ☐ Star anise (3 whole)
- ☐ Black tea bags (5)
- ☐ Whole milk (2 cups)
- ☐ Vanilla extract (1 tbsp.)
- ☐ Optional: Ground nutmeg

Preparation Guidelines:

1. Use a mortar and pestle or spice grinder to combine the peppercorns and cardamom pods until the aromas are released.
2. Prepare a saucepan of water. Once it is boiling, add in the cardamom mixture, cinnamon sticks, honey, cloves, ginger, and star anise. Simmer for about five minutes or to your liking Transfer it to a cool burner and add the tea bags. Place a lid on the pot to steep for five minutes.
3. Warm the milk in a small pan.
4. Strain the tea to discard the spices and tea bags.
5. Pour the hot milk and the vanilla into mugs with a dusting of nutmeg as desired.

Hot Chocolate

Servings: 4 | **Difficulty**: Super Easy | **Time**: 15 min

Nutrition per Serving:

- Calories: 249
- Carbohydrates: 36 grams
- Protein: 9 grams
- Fat: 8 grams
- Sat. Fats: 5 grams
- Sugars: 30 grams
- Fiber: 0 grams

Ingredients Needed:

- ☐ Miniature marshmallows (1.5 cups)
- ☐ Sugar (8 tsp.)
- ☐ Baking cocoa (4 tsp.)
- ☐ 2% milk (4 cups)
- ☐ Vanilla extract (1 tsp.)

Preparation Guidelines:

1. Prepare a saucepan using the medium temperature setting. Mix in the milk, vanilla, cocoa, and sugar. Simmer for about eight minutes.
2. Transfer to a cool burner and add the vanilla to serve in a warm mug.

Iced Coconut Mocha Macchiato

Servings: 1 | **Difficulty**: Easy | **Time**: 10 min

Nutrition per Serving:

- Calories: 582
- Protein: 6 grams
- Fat: 51 grams
- Sat. Fats: 44 grams
- Carbohydrates: 30 grams
- Sugars: 13 grams
- Fiber: 1 gram

Ingredients Needed:

- ☐ Chocolate sauce (2 tbsp.)
- ☐ Expresso (1.5 oz.)
- ☐ Coconut milk (1 cup)

Preparation Guidelines:

1. For the espresso, you can also use one teaspoon of instant espresso and a few ounces of hot water or just use four ounces of strong coffee.
2. Layer the chocolate sauce, espresso, and milk.
3. Toss in the ice.
4. Garnish it using whipped cream and caramel or chocolate sauce.
5. In case you are out of espresso, use a cup of regular or leftover coffee.

S'mores Frappuccino

Servings: 1 | **Difficulty**: Easy | **Time**: 10 min

Nutrition per Serving:

- Calories: 623
- Protein: 10 grams
- Fat: 21 grams
- Sat. Fats: 12 grams
- Carbohydrates: 97 grams
- Sugars: 74 grams
- Fiber: 2 grams

Ingredients Needed:

- ☐ Marshmallow fluff (2 tbsp.)
- ☐ Chocolate syrup (1 tbsp.)
- ☐ Ice (1 cup)
- ☐ Milk (.5 cup)
- ☐ Vanilla ice cream (1 cup)
- ☐ Cold coffee (.25 cup)
- ☐ Torani S'mores syrup (2 tbsp.)
- ☐ Whipped cream (1 tbsp.)
- ☐ Graham cracker (1)

Preparation Guidelines:

1. Measure and add the milk, ice, coffee, ice cream, and syrup into a blender.
2. Mix and pour the fluff into the glass. Top it off using a portion of whipped cream and a drizzle of syrup and crushed crackers.
3. You can also swap the ice with a frozen banana and mix with other fixings to enjoy another healthier version.

Salted Caramel Mocha

Servings: 6 | **Difficulty**: Easy | **Time**: 20 min

Nutrition per Serving - 1 cup of coffee + 2 tbsp. whipped cream:

- Calories: 220
- Carbohydrates: 19 grams
- Protein: 3 grams
- Fat: 14 grams
- Sat. Fats: 9 grams
- Sugars: 16 grams
- Fiber: 1 gram

Ingredients Needed:
- ☐ Heavy whipping cream (.5 cup)
- ☐ Confectioner's sugar (1 tbsp.)
- ☐ Vanilla extract (1 tsp. - divided)
- ☐ Dutch-processed cocoa (.25 cup)
- ☐ Half & Half cream (1.5 cups)
- ☐ Strong hot brewed coffee (4 cups)
- ☐ Caramel flavoring syrup (.5 cup)
- ☐ Butterscotch-caramel ice cream topping
- ☐ Also Needed: 3-quart slow cooker

Preparation Guidelines:

1. Whisk the whipping cream until it begins to thicken. Mix in the confectioners' sugar and 1/2 teaspoon vanilla, beating to create stiff peaks.
2. Prepare a saucepan using the medium temperature setting.
3. Whisk the Half & Half and cocoa until smooth. Warm it until it's bubbly.
4. Whisk in the caramel syrup, coffee, and rest of the vanilla. Garnish each serving with whipped cream and a drizzle of the butterscotch topping.
5. Prepare the whipped cream as directed. Whisk the cocoa, half-and-half, coffee, caramel syrup, and remaining vanilla in the cooker. Securely close the lid to cook for two to three hours or until heated thoroughly. Serve as directed.

Chapter 11: Subway™ Specialties

Breakfast

BMT Sandwich

Servings: 1 | **Difficulty**: Easy | **Time**: 30 min

Nutrition per Serving:
- Calories: 725
- Carbohydrates: 56 grams
- Protein: 36 grams
- Fat: 41 grams
- Sat. Fats: 15 grams
- Sugars: 15 grams
- Fiber: 8 grams

Ingredients Needed:

Fixings: 2 slices each:
- ☐ Bread
- ☐ Pepperoni
- ☐ Ham
- ☐ Salami
- ☐ Provolone cheese
- ☐ Onions

Other Toppings:
- ☐ Shredded lettuce (.25 cup)
- ☐ Roasted jalapenos (1 tbsp.)
- ☐ Tomatoes (3 slices)
- ☐ Black pepper (1 tbsp.)
- ☐ Mayo (1 tbsp.)
- ☐ Sandwich spread (1 tbsp.)

Preparation Guidelines:

1. Prepare the loaf of bread by vertically slicing it in half.
2. Toss the bread with the lettuce, meat slices, jalapenos, onions, and tomatoes.
3. Garnish it with may and the sandwich spread.
4. Enjoy your delightful BMT copycat!

Subway™ Bread Recipe

Servings: 8 or ½ of a bun - Total of 4 - 9-inch sub buns | **Difficulty**: Medium | **Time**: 2 hours

Nutrition per Serving:

- Calories: 244
- Carbohydrates: 38.3 grams
- Protein: 5.8 grams
- Fat: 7.6 grams
- Sat. Fats: grams
- Sugars: 1.7 grams

Ingredients Needed:

- ☐ Yeast (1 tbsp.)
- ☐ Warm water @ 110° Fahrenheit (1 cup)
- ☐ Salt (1.5 tsp.)
- ☐ Sugar (1 tbsp.)
- ☐ A-P flour (2.5-2.75 cups)
- ☐ Olive oil (4 tbsp.)
- ☐ Also Needed: Stand mixer & dough hook

Preparation Guidelines:

1. When it's time, warm the oven to reach 350° Fahrenheit. Prepare and set aside a cookie sheet lined with a layer of parchment baking paper.
2. Combine the oil, water, yeast, sugar, and salt into the bowl of a stand mixer, add. Wait for about five minutes for the yeast to work its magic.
3. Sift in one cup of flour and combine using the dough hook for three to five minutes.
4. Sift and work in another cup of flour.
5. Continue adding increments of ¼ cup of the flour until a soft dough is formed. Only work the dough for eight minutes - total.

6. When the dough is formed, scoop it onto a lightly floured surface and knead until smooth. Shape the dough into a ball and return it to the bowl. Cover the bowl with plastic wrap and allow the dough to rise for half an hour.
7. At that point, scoop it out onto a floured surface and divide it into four portions. Roll each piece of dough into a long skinny loaf that is (nine to ten inches long).
8. Arrange the loaves on the baking tray. Continue the process with the remainder of the dough, leaving at least two inches between each loaf on the pan.
9. Use a layer of greased plastic to cover the loaves while you wait for them to rise in a warm space until doubled in size (one hour).
10. When the loaves are ready, bake them for 25 minutes.
11. When the loaves come out of the oven, generously grease the tops using butter. Cover them with a dish towel to cool for at least an hour.
12. When they are cooled, prepare as desired. Yummy!

Subway ™ Sweet Onion Chicken Teriyaki Sandwiches

Servings: 4 | **Difficulty**: Easy | **Time**: 20 min

Nutrition per Serving:

- Calories: 610
- Protein: 51 grams
- Fat Content: 20 grams
- Sat. Fats: 6 grams
- Carbohydrates: 57 grams
- Sugars: 13 grams
- Fibers: 2 grams

Ingredients Needed:

- ☐ Grilled chicken breast strips - frozen (1 lb.)
- ☐ Teriyaki glaze (3 tbsp.)
- ☐ Soft hoagie rolls - halved (4)
- ☐ Provolone cheese (4 slices - 0.7 oz. each - cut into halves)
- ☐ Baby spinach (1.5 cups)
- ☐ Diced red onion (2 tbsp.)
- ☐ Sweet onion dressing (.25 cup)

Preparation Guidelines:

1. Toss the chicken into a 12-inch skillet. Cover the pan and heat using medium heat 10 to 12 minutes, occasionally stirring until thoroughly heated.
2. Uncover and add the teriyaki glaze, stirring continuously until well coated. Remove the mixture from heat.
3. Divide the chicken among bottom halves of rolls.
4. Top with cheese, spinach, onion, and dressing.

Lunch

Orchard Chicken Salad

Servings: 4 | **Difficulty**: Easy | **Time**: 25 min

Nutrition per Serving:
- Calories: 402
- Carbohydrates: 30 grams
- Protein: 33 grams
- Fat: 16 grams
- Sat. Fats: 3 grams
- Sugars: 21 grams
- Fiber: 3 grams

Ingredients Needed:
- ☐ Cooked chicken breast (3 cups)
- ☐ Red apple - ex. Honey crisp (1)
- ☐ Granny Smith apple (1)
- ☐ Chopped celery (.5 cup)
- ☐ Cherry juice - infused craisins (.5 cup)
- ☐ Light mayo (1 cup)
- ☐ Pepper & salt (as desired)

Preparation Guidelines:

1. Chop the apples in a mixing container and sprinkle with one tablespoon of juice.
2. Chop and add the celery, chicken, and Craisins, mixing thoroughly.
3. Lastly, add in the salt, pepper, and mayo.
4. Marinate the fixings in the fridge about one hour before it's serving time.

Dinner

Meatball Sub

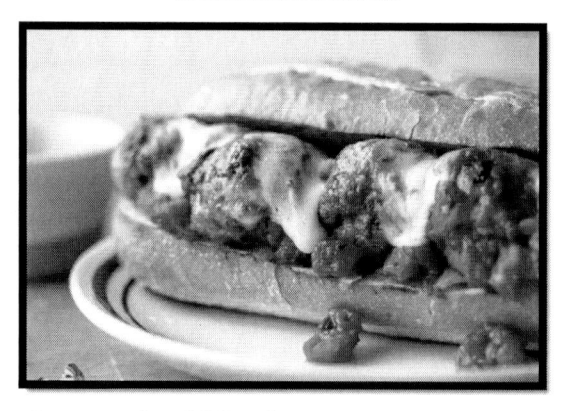

Servings: 4 | **Difficulty**: Easy | **Time**: 40 min

Nutrition per Serving:

- Calories: 1453
- Carbohydrates: 93 grams
- Protein: 53 grams
- Fat: 97 grams
- Sat. Fats: 46 grams
- Sugars: 56 grams
- Fiber: 9 grams

Ingredients Needed:

- ☐ Plain bread (1 slice)
- ☐ Milk (.25 cup)
- ☐ Ground beef combo - veal - beef & pork (1.25 lb.)
- ☐ Lightly whisked egg (1 large)
- ☐ Finely grated parmesan cheese (.5 cup - divided)
- ☐ Freshly minced parsley (2 tbsp.)
- ☐ Finely minced garlic (.5 tsp.)
- ☐ Kosher salt (.5 tsp./as needed)
- ☐ Freshly cracked pepper (as desired)
- ☐ Olive oil (2 tbsp. for sautéing)

- ☐ Marinara sauce (4 cups)
- ☐ Italian bread (4 slices - sliced lengthwise/1 loaf)
- ☐ Shredded mozzarella cheese (1 cup)

Preparation Guidelines:

1. Warm the oven to 350° Fahrenheit.
2. Slice the bread and place them in a bowl with the milk. Stir to mix and wait for five minutes until the majority of the liquid is absorbed. Remove the excess milk and shred the bread to bits.
3. Toss the meat in a mixing container with ¼ cup of parmesan, the soaked bread, garlic, parsley, and ½ teaspoon of salt and pepper. Mix and shape into two-inch meatballs.
4. Bake the meatballs on a lightly greased baking tray (15 min.).
5. Pour and warm the marinara sauce in a medium pot using the med-low temperature setting. Add the meatballs and simmer for about ten more minutes.
6. Meanwhile, prepare the rolls either soft or toasted. Open them up, spritz lightly with oil, and toast them on a hot skillet as desired.
7. Adjust the oven setting to broil.
8. Place the meatballs with the sauce into a shallow baking dish (single-layered).
9. Sprinkle with mozzarella and rest of the parmesan.
10. Bake for about one or two minutes until the cheese is melted.
11. Scoop the meatballs onto the rolls and serve steaming hot.

Dessert

Chewy Peanut Butter Cookies

Servings: 27 cookies | **Difficulty**: Very Easy | **Time**: 27-30 min

Nutrition per Serving:

- Calories: 211
- Carbohydrates: 23 grams
- Protein: 4 grams
- Fat: 12 grams
- Sat. Fats: 4 grams
- Sugars: 14 grams
- Fiber: 1 gram

Ingredients Needed:

The Dough:
- ☐ Peanut butter (1 cup)
- ☐ Shortening (.5 cup)
- ☐ Butter (4 oz./1 stick)
- ☐ Brown sugar (1 cup)
- ☐ Granulated sugar (.75 cup)
- ☐ Eggs (2)
- ☐ Flour (2 cups)
- ☐ Baking soda (2 tsp.)
- ☐ Salt (1 tsp.)
- ☐ Optional: Chopped peanuts (.25 cup)

Preparation Guidelines:

1. Cream both types of butter with the shortening and sugar for two minutes until it's fluffy.
2. Whisk and add in the eggs, mixing with the dry ones. Fold in the nuts.
3. Scoop the dough using a 1.5-inch scoop, placing them onto a baking tray about two inches apart.
4. Bake for 11 minutes.

White Chocolate Raspberry Cookies

Servings: 36 | **Difficulty**: Easy | **Time**: 25 min

Nutrition per Serving:

- Calories: 115
- Carbohydrates: 9 grams
- Protein: 1 gram
- Fat: 7 grams
- Sat. Fats: 4 grams
- Sugars: 5 grams

Ingredients Needed:
- ☐ Unchilled cream cheese (4 oz.)
- ☐ Softened butter (.5 cup)
- ☐ Shortening (2 tbsp.)
- ☐ Brown sugar (.5 cup)
- ☐ Eggs (2)
- ☐ Jiffy raspberry muffin mix (2 - 7 oz. boxes)
- ☐ All-Purpose flour (.75 cup)
- ☐ White chocolate chips (1.5 cups)

Preparation Guidelines:
1. Beat the shortening, cream cheese, butter, and brown sugar in an over-sized mixing container.
2. Once mixed, mix in the eggs - one at a time.
3. Combine the flour and muffin mix with the white chips, stirring until they are fully incorporated.
4. Chill the dough for a minimum of half an hour.
5. Warm the oven to 350° Fahrenheit and prepare a baking tray using a spritz of cooking oil spray.
6. Scoop the mix onto the prepared pans and bake for 10 to 12 minutes.
7. Note: Keep the dough chilled during preparation.

Chapter 12: Wendy's™ Specialties

Brunch

Artisan Bacon Egg Sandwich

Servings: 4 | **Difficulty**: Easy | **Time**: 20 min

Nutrition per Serving:

- Calories: 461
- Protein: 19 grams
- Fat: 27 grams
- Sat. Fats: 13 grams
- Carbohydrates: 32 grams
- Sugars: 6 grams
- Fiber: 2 grams

Ingredients Needed:

- ☐ Sour cream (.5 cup)
- ☐ Bread slices (8)
- ☐ Green onions (4)
- ☐ American cheese (4 slices)
- ☐ Hard-boiled eggs (2)
- ☐ Bacon strips (8)
- ☐ Unchilled butter (2 tbsp.)

Preparation Guidelines:

1. Chop the onion and slice the boiled eggs into ¼-inch slices.
2. Spread a portion of sour cream over four bread slices. Top each one using green onions, eggs, cheese, bacon, and rest of the bread.
3. Spread the outsides of sandwiches with butter.
4. Toast the sandwiches until golden brown and cheese are melted (2-3 min. per side).

Baconator

Servings: 4 | **Difficulty**: Easy | **Time**: 30 min

Nutrition per Serving:
- Calories: 472
- Carbohydrates: 27 grams
- Protein: 33 grams
- Fat: 25 grams
- Sat. Fats: 10 grams
- Sugars: 7 grams
- Fiber: 1 gram

Ingredients Needed:
- ☐ Onion (2 tbsp.)
- ☐ Ketchup (2 tbsp.)
- ☐ Garlic (1 clove)
- ☐ Sugar (1 tsp.)
- ☐ Worcestershire sauce (1 tsp.)
- ☐ Cider vinegar (.25 tsp.)
- ☐ Steak sauce (1 tsp.)
- ☐ Ground beef (1 lb.)
- ☐ Burger buns (4 toasted)
- ☐ Bacon strips (8 cooked)
- ☐ Sharp cheddar cheese (4 slices)

Optional Garnishes:
- ☐ Lettuce leaves
- ☐ Onion slices
- ☐ Sliced pickles
- ☐ Tomato slices

Preparation Guidelines:

1. Finely chop the garlic and onion.
2. Combine the onion, ketchup, sugar, Worcestershire sauce, steak sauce, and vinegar. Add the beef, mixing and shaping it into four patties.
3. Grill the burgers, covered - using the medium temperature setting for four to seven minutes per side (160° Fahrenheit internal temp).
4. Top the meat with cheese and grill until the cheese is melted.
5. Serve the burgers on buns with bacon and toppings as desired.

Grilled Asiago Ranch Chicken Club

Servings: 4 | **Difficulty**: Quick & Easy | **Time**: 25 min

Nutrition per Serving:

- Calories: 410
- Protein: 34 grams
- Fat: 17 grams
- Sat. Fats: 6 grams
- Carbohydrates: 29 grams
- Fiber: 3 grams
- Sugars: 9 grams

Ingredients Needed:
- ☐ Honey (1 tbsp.)
- ☐ Reduced-fat mayo (.25 cup)
- ☐ Dijon mustard (1 tbsp.)
- ☐ Montreal steak seasoning (.5 tsp.)
- ☐ Chicken breast halves (4 @ 4 oz. each)
- ☐ Swiss cheese (4 slices)
- ☐ Split whole-wheat burger buns (4 - split)
- ☐ Bacon slices (2 crumbled & cooked)
- ☐ Optional: Lettuce leaves & sliced tomatoes

Preparation Guidelines:

1. Whisk the honey, mayonnaise, and mustard. Use a sharp knife to discard the skin and bones from the chicken, and a meat mallet to pound it into a ½-inch thickness.
2. Dust the chicken with the steak seasoning and grill it with the lid on, using the medium temperature setting or broil it about four inches from heat (four to six min. per side).
3. Sprinkle the cheese over the top during the last minute of the cooking cycle.
4. Grill the buns (medium heat) cut side down, until toasted, 30-60 seconds.
5. Serve the chicken on buns with the mayo mixture, lettuce, bacon, and tomato.

Power Mediterranean Chicken Salad

Servings: 4 | **Difficulty**: Easy | **Time**: 25 min

Nutrition per Serving:

- Calories: 341
- Carbohydrates: 27 grams
- Protein: 19 grams
- Fat: 19 grams
- Sat. Fats: 3 grams
- Fiber: 4 grams
- Sugars: 3 grams

Ingredients Needed:

- ☐ Water - divided (1.5 cups + 2 tbsp.)
- ☐ Rinsed quinoa (.75 cup)
- ☐ Plain yogurt (2 tbsp.)
- ☐ Sriracha chili sauce (1 tsp.)
- ☐ Mayonnaise (1 tbsp.)
- ☐ Crumbled feta cheese (.25 cup)
- ☐ Cucumber (1 medium - seeded)
- ☐ Fresh parsley (.75 cup)
- ☐ Green onions (2)
- ☐ Olive oil (.25 cup)
- ☐ Greek seasoning (.75 tsp.)
- ☐ Lemon juice (3 tbsp.)
- ☐ Chicken breast strips (grilled & ready-to-use/6 oz. pkg.)
- ☐ Tomato (1 medium)

Preparation Guidelines:

1. Finely chop the onions, tomato, cucumber, and parsley.
2. Boil 1.5 cups of water and add the quinoa. Use the medium temperature setting and simmer, covered until liquid is absorbed, 12-15 minutes.
3. For the dressing, place remaining water, yogurt, mayonnaise, chili sauce, and cheese in a blender or food processor. Cover with the top and process until blended.
4. Rinse the cooked quinoa in a strainer with cold water; drain well.
5. Toss the quinoa with cucumber, parsley, green onions, oil, lemon juice, and Greek seasoning in a serving dish. Top with chicken, tomato, and dressing.

Lunch

Cheesy Stuffed Baked Potato

Servings: 6 | **Difficulty**: Easy | **Time**: 1 hour 45 min

Nutrition per Serving:

- Calories: 416
- Protein: 9 grams
- Fat: 26 grams
- Sat. Fats: 17 grams
- Carbohydrates: 36 grams
- Fiber: 3 grams
- Sugars: 4 grams

Ingredients Needed:

- ☐ Large baking potatoes (3 large/1 lb. each)
- ☐ Optional: Canola oil (1.5 tsp.)
- ☐ Green onions (.5 cup)
- ☐ Half & Half cream (.5 cup)
- ☐ Cubed butter - divided (.5 cup)
- ☐ Sour cream (.5 cup)
- ☐ White pepper (.5 tsp.)
- ☐ Salt (1 tsp.)
- ☐ Paprika (as desired)
- ☐ Shredded cheddar cheese (1 cup)

Preparation Guidelines:

1. Scrub each of the potatoes, poking them with a fork, and prepping with oil. Warm the oven and bake them at 400° Fahrenheit for 50 minutes to 1 hour 15 minutes until they are tender.
2. Once they are cooled, slice each potato in half (lengthwise). Use a spoon to remove the pulp from the potato skin.
3. Slice and sauté the onions in the ¼ cup butter until tender.
4. Stuff the Potatoes: Mash the potato pulp and stir in the sour cream, cream, onion mixture, pepper, and salt. Blend in the cheese and prepare each of the shells.
5. Arrange them onto a baking tray. Melt in the rest of the butter and drizzle over potatoes. Sprinkle with paprika to your liking.
6. Bake at 375 °Fahrenheit for 20 minutes and serve.

Chili - Slow-Cooked

Servings: 10/2.5 quarts | **Difficulty**: Easy | **Time**: 8 hours 20 min

Nutrition per Serving - 1 cup portion:

- Calories: 260
- Carbohydrates: 23 grams
- Protein: 25 grams
- Fat: 8 grams
- Sat. Fats: 3 grams
- Sugars: 6 grams
- Fiber: 7 grams

Ingredients Needed:

- ☐ 90% lean ground beef (2 lb.)
- ☐ Kidney beans (2 - 16 oz. cans)
- ☐ Undrained diced tomatoes (2 - 14.5 oz. cans)
- ☐ Tomato sauce (8oz. can)
- ☐ Medium onions (2)
- ☐ Garlic (2 cloves)
- ☐ Green pepper (1)
- ☐ Black pepper & salt (1 tsp. each)
- ☐ Chili powder (2 tbsp.)

Optional Toppings:
- ☐ Thinly sliced onions
- ☐ Shredded cheddar cheese
- ☐ Also Needed: 5-quart slow cooker

Preparation Guidelines:

1. Add and cook the beef in a skillet (medium temp) until it's no longer pink and drain. Transfer it to the cooker.
2. Chop/mince the onions, peppers, and garlic. Rinse and drain the beans. Add everything but the onions and cheese.
3. Securely close the lid and set the timer using the low setting for eight to ten hours.
4. If desired, top individual servings with cheese and green onions.

Dave's Single

Servings: 4 | **Difficulty**: Super Easy | **Time**: 25 min

Nutrition per Serving - no toppings:

- Calories: 429
- Carbohydrates: 32 grams
- Protein: 28 grams
- Fat: 20 grams
- Sat. Fats: 6 grams
- Fiber: 1 gram
- Sugars: 3 grams

Ingredients Needed:

- ☐ Olive oil (1 tbsp.)
- ☐ Seasoned breadcrumbs (.5 cup)
- ☐ Large egg (1)
- ☐ Black pepper & salt (.5 tsp. each)
- ☐ Ground beef (1 lb.)
- ☐ Split sesame seed burger buns (4)
- ☐ Optional: Garnish as desired

Preparation Guidelines:

1. Whisk the egg, salt, and pepper. Mix it in with the breadcrumbs and beef, shaping it into four ½-inch-thick patties.
2. Light spritz both sides of the patty using oil before arranging them on the grill. Set the grill using the medium temperature setting.
3. Grill the burger with the lid on for four to five minutes on each side as desired.
4. Serve on buns with the desired toppings.

Spicy Chicken Nuggets

Servings: 6 | **Difficulty**: Very Easy | **Time**: 30 min

Nutrition per Serving:

- Calories: 371
- Protein: 29 grams
- Fat: 22 grams
- Sat. Fats: 10 grams
- Carbohydrates: 13 grams
- Sugars: 1 gram
- Fiber: 1 gram

Ingredients Needed:

- ☐ Panko breadcrumbs (1.5 cups)
- ☐ Parmesan cheese (1.5 cups - grated)
- ☐ Optional: Ground chipotle pepper (.5 tsp.)
- ☐ Butter (.25 cup)
- ☐ Chicken thighs (1.5 lb. chopped into 1.5-inch chunks)
- ☐ Also Needed: 15x10x1-inch baking pan

Preparation Guidelines:

1. Warm the oven at 400 °Fahrenheit.
2. In a shallow bowl, combine the breadcrumbs, cheese, and chipotle pepper.
3. Melt and add the butter in another preparation container.
4. Dip the pieces of chicken in butter and crumb mixture, patting to help the coating adhere.
5. Place chicken on the baking tray with a sprinkle of the crumb mixture. Set a timer to bake it until no longer pink (20-25 min.).
6. Serve with your favorite sides.

Dinner

Apple Pecan Chicken Salad

Servings: 6 | **Difficulty**: Super Easy | **Time**: 30 min

Nutrition per Serving:

- Calories: 306
- Protein: 17 grams
- Fat: 19 grams
- Sat. Fats: 3 grams
- Carbohydrates: 20 grams
- Sugars: 12 grams
- Fiber: 4 grams

Ingredients Needed:

The Vinaigrette:
- ☐ Balsamic vinegar (.25 cup)
- ☐ Orange juice (.25 cup)
- ☐ Olive oil (.25 cup)
- ☐ Lemon juice (2 tbsp.)
- ☐ Brown sugar (1 tbsp.)
- ☐ Soy sauce (2 tbsp.)
- ☐ Dijon mustard (1 tbsp.)
- ☐ Optional: Curry powder (.5 tsp.)
- ☐ Salt (.5 tsp.)
- ☐ Black pepper (.25 tsp.)
- ☐ Ground ginger (.25 tsp.)

The Salad:
- ☐ Shredded chicken (2 cups)
- ☐ Apples (2 medium)
- ☐ Red onion (.5 cup)
- ☐ Mixed salad greens (10 cups)
- ☐ Toasted chopped walnuts (.5 cup)

Preparation Guidelines:

1. Cook and shred the chicken. Thinly slice the onions and chop the apples.
2. Prepare a shallow pan to toast the nuts. Set a timer to bake at 350° Fahrenheit for five to ten minutes. You can also cook it in a skillet using the low-temperature setting until lightly browned, stirring intermittently.
3. Whisk the vinaigrette fixings until thoroughly mixed. Add chicken, apples, and onions, tossing to coat.
4. Just before serving, tear and place greens on a large serving plate and top with the chicken mixture. Sprinkle with walnuts.

Taco Salad

Servings: 2 | **Difficulty**: Easy | **Time**: 25 min

Nutrition per Serving:

- Calories: 469
- Carbohydrates: 25 grams
- Protein: 32 grams
- Fat: 28 grams
- Sat. Fats: 12 grams
- Sugars: 5 grams
- Fiber: 4 grams

Ingredients Needed:
- ☐ Ground beef (.5 lb.)
- ☐ Bean dip (.33 cup)
- ☐ Chili powder (1 tsp.)
- ☐ Salt (.25 tsp.)
- ☐ Diced tomatoes (1 cup canned + 2 tbsp. liquid)
- ☐ Chopped lettuce (2 cups)
- ☐ Shredded cheddar cheese (.5 cup)
- ☐ Sliced green onions (2)
- ☐ Sliced ripe olives (2 tbsp.)
- ☐ Corn chips (.5 cup)

Preparation Guidelines:

1. Prepare a skillet using the medium temperature setting. Toss in the beef to cook until it's no longer pink and drain.
2. Mix in the bean dip, chili powder, salt, and tomato liquid. Transfer the pan to a cool burner.
3. Combine the tomatoes, lettuce, cheese, onions, and olives in a large salad container.
4. Add the beef mixture, tossing to coat. Top with the chips and serve right away.

Dessert

<u>Double Chocolate Chip Cookies</u>

Servings: 4.5 dozen cookies | **Difficulty**: Easy | **Time**: 30 min

Nutrition per Serving - 2 cookies each:

- Calories: 238
- Protein: 2 grams
- Fat: 13 grams
- Sat. Fats: 8 grams
- Carbohydrates: 31 grams
- Fiber: 1 gram

Ingredients Needed:

- ☐ Unchilled butter (1.25 cup)
- ☐ Sugar (2 cups)
- ☐ Unchilled eggs (2 large eggs)
- ☐ Vanilla extract (2 tsp.)
- ☐ Baking cocoa (.75 cup)
- ☐ Salt (.5 tsp.)
- ☐ A-P flour (2 cups)
- ☐ Baking soda (1 tsp.)
- ☐ Dark chocolate semisweet chocolate chips (2 cups)

Preparation Guidelines:

1. Warm the oven to 350 ° Fahrenheit
2. Cream the butter with the sugar until fluffy. Blend in the vanilla and eggs.
3. In another container, whisk the baking soda, cocoa, flour, and salt. Gradually, add it to the creamed mixture. Stir in chips.
4. Drop by teaspoonfuls onto lightly greased baking trays. Bake them for eight to ten minutes (do not overbake). Cool on the pans for one minute. Lastly, place them onto wire racks to cool.

Frosty Time

Servings: 1 | **Difficulty**: Super Easy | **Time**: 5 min

Nutrition per Serving:

- Calories: 520
- Carbohydrates: 84 grams
- Fat: 14 grams
- Sat. Fats: 8 grams
- Sugars: 66 grams
- Fiber: 3 grams
- Protein: 17 grams

Ingredients Needed:

- ☐ Chocolate milk ice cubes (16)
- ☐ Cool Whip/whipped cream (1 cup)
- ☐ Sweetened condensed milk (1 tbsp.)

Preparation Guidelines:

1. Freeze the chocolate milk in an ice cube tray to freeze ahead of frosty time.
2. Toss each of the fixings in a blender.
3. Pulse until the mixture is creamy smooth. Scrape the sides as needed and serve in a frosty cup!

Conclusion

I hope you have enjoyed all of the selections in *Copycat Recipes*. I hope it was informative and provided you with all of the tools you need to achieve your goals, making the most delicious 'take-out' in your kitchen. The next step is to gather the necessary ingredients to make delicious meals and treats.

You will also need to know how to properly store your masterpiece selections. For meals that are scheduled to be eaten at least three days after cooking, freezing is a great option. Freezing food is safe and convenient, but it doesn't work for every type of meal. You can also freeze the ingredients for a slow cooker meal and then dump out the container into the slow cooker and leave it there. This saves a lot of time and means you can pre-prep meals up to one to two months in advance.

You must also know the proper ways to reheat your meals. Most people opt to microwave their meals for warming, but you can use any other conventional heating source in your kitchen as well. However, you have to be careful with microwaving because over-cooking can cause food to taste bad.

To combat this, cook your food in one-minute intervals and check on it between each minute. You can also help your food cook more evenly and quickly but keeping your meat cut into small pieces when you cook it. You should never put food directly from the freezer into the microwave. Let your frozen food thaw first when it's possible.

Food reheating and prep safety will become second nature over time. However, mistakes do happen, and as such, it's best to cook for short periods rather than longer ones, so you have less of a risk of making a mistake and needing to scrap everything you have prepared for that substantial amount of time. While it is a lot and seems complicated, meal prepping is the best way to set yourself up for success using your delicious copycat recipes. Make the meals using double the products and adjust the times; that is all it is to it!

Don't store hot food in the fridge. Keep your refrigerator at the proper temperature (should be below 40º Fahrenheit). If your refrigerator is warmer than this, it promotes the growth of bacteria. Any drastic temperature changes will cause condensation to form on the food items. You need to let your prepared food cool down in the open air - before putting it in a container and closing the lid. The increased moisture levels can open the door to bacteria growth.

There are some other things you have to consider when freezing your meals. You should always label your container with the date that you put it in the freezer. You also need to double-check that your bottles, jars, or bags are each sealed tightly. If your containers aren't air-tight, your food will become freezer burnt and need to be trashed.

I hope these additional suggestions will make your Copycat Recipes a treasured item in your digital library. Why not get started right now? Have fun, and enjoy the time and money saved cooking at home!

If you found this book useful in any way, a review on Amazon is always appreciated! Thank you :)

Copycat Italian Recipes

Stacy Earls

Introduction

Congratulations on purchasing Copycat Recipes, and thank you for doing so!
Welcome to the world of exotic and spicy foods provided with the Italian cuisine.
You will indulge in the most flavorful ingredients, deliciously portrayed with each authentic Italian dish that is duplicated in your new cookbook of Copycat Recipes. Traditional products are essential for the flavors of Italy, which, at their best, are based on seasonality and locality.

You will be using extra-virgin olive oil, which is the blueprint of most Italian cooking, whether you are frying, braising, or drizzling it over your veggies; it will become heavenly.
Onions and garlic are two widely used produce items, but the green vegetables are frequently in the #1 slot. You won't find an Italian kitchen without a supply of balsamic vinegar.

Fish is considered a staple on the Italian diet, whether you have a fresh catch, purchase it from the market, or canned in oil. You will notice many of the recipes use a fabulous variety of shrimp, tilapia, and many others.
Cured meats are also plentiful.
The Italian culture believes it is vital to preserve the meats by making pork into salami and sausage, using the oil from olives, wine from grapes, and veggies into pickled delicacies.

You will enjoy each one of the delightful options provided in restaurants, including:

- *Biaggi's Ristorante Italiano Restaurant*
- *Carrabba's Italian Grill*
- *Olive Garden*
- *Original Sicilian Pasta Co.*
- *Pasta House Company*
- *Fazoli's*
- *Romano's Macaroni Grill*
- *NYC Restaurants*
- *The Old Spaghetti Factory*
- *Zio's Italian Kitchen*

I hope you will enjoy each of the delicious recipes in your home's comfort and feel delighted that you can save the tip for a night out of movies or dancing!

Wait a second! To thank you for your purchase, I want to give you a free Special Chapter about Best Italian Recipes! Just a quick click on the link below! Thanks and happy reading!

Let's Get Started!

Chapter 1: Olive Garden Specialities

Brunch Options
<u>*Angry Alfredo With Chicken*</u>

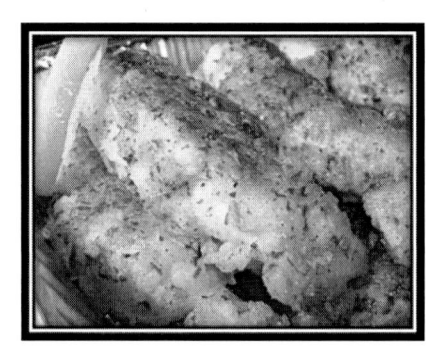

Servings: 4 | **Difficulty**: Easy | **Time**: 30-35 minutes

Ingredients Needed:

The Sauce:
- Butter (4 oz.)
- Heavy cream (1 cup)
- Fresh parmesan cheese (.5 cup - grated)
- Garlic powder (.5 tsp.)
- Red pepper chili flakes (.25 tsp.)

The Chicken:
- Olive oil (1 tbsp.)
- Chicken breast (8 oz.)
- Black pepper & salt (to your liking)

The Topping: Mozzarella cheese (.5 cup)

Preparation Guidelines:
1. Prepare a saucepan using the med-high temperature setting.
2. Pour in the heavy cream. Once bubbling, mix in the cheese and stir until the sauce thickens. Adjust the temperature setting to simmer and add the crushed red peppers and garlic powder.
3. Season the chicken with pepper and salt.
4. Warm a cast-iron skillet using the med-high setting to warm the oil. Cook the chicken for five to seven minutes until the edges of the chicken begin to turn white.
5. Turn the chicken over and continue to cook until done (5-7 min.). Set aside the chicken a few minutes (2-3) to rest.
6. Warm the oven using the broil setting. Slice the chicken into bite-sized pieces.
7. Combine the Alfredo sauce and the chicken and dump it into a one-quart casserole dish. Top with mozzarella cheese and broil until browned as desired.

Baked Parmesan Shrimp

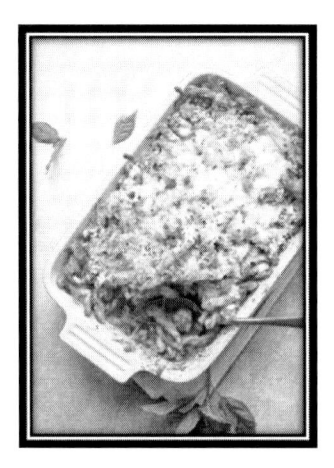

Servings: 4 | **Difficulty**: Super-Easy | **Time**: 20-25 minutes

Ingredients Needed:
- Pasta (your favorite - 8 oz. pkg.)
- Butter (4 oz.)
- Parmesan cheese (8 oz.)
- Heavy cream (1 pint)
- Shrimp (8 oz.)
- Roma tomato (1 in small pieces)
- Chopped parsley (2 tsp.)
- Breadcrumbs (2 tbsp.)
- Parmesan cheese (2 tsp.)
- Melted butter (1 tbsp.)

Preparation Guidelines:
1. Cook, peel, and remove the veins of the shrimp. Cook the pasta per the package details (8-12 min.)
2. Warm the oven at 350° Fahrenheit.
3. Prepare a medium saucepan to melt the butter with the heavy cream. Measure and add in the parmesan and stir until it's melted, adding pepper and salt as desired.
4. Toss the pasta in a dish and mix it with the sauce. Add it to two to three small casserole dishes.
5. Combine the melted butter, breadcrumbs, and parmesan in a mixing container, and add to the top of the casserole dishes. Add several pieces of shrimp on each one and bake until it's thoroughly heated.
6. Garnish with parsley and a few chopped tomatoes.

Tortellini al Forno

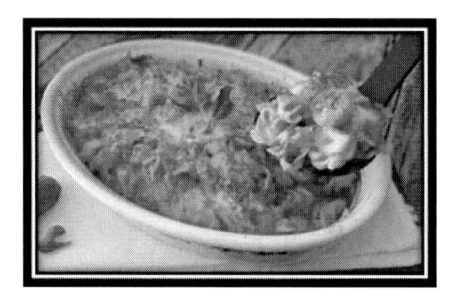

Servings: 4 | **Difficulty**: Super-Easy | **Time**: 15-20 minutes

Ingredients Needed:
- Tortellini (9 oz.)
- Butter (6 tbsp.)
- Heavy cream (.5 cup)
- Grated parmesan cheese (.5 cup)
- Crispy bacon (1 oz.)
- Sliced scallions (1 tbsp.)

Preparation Guidelines:
1. Prepare the tortellini per the package insert (approx. 7 min.).
2. Use a small saucepan (medium temperature setting) to warm the heavy cream and melt the butter. Once the mixture starts to bubble slightly, mix in the parmesan cheese until it melts completely.
3. Arrange eight to ten pieces of tortellini in each dish. Add the melted cheese, sliced scallions, and crumbled bacon over the tortellini to serve.

Dinner Options
Baked Tilapia & Shrimp

Servings: 4 | **Difficulty**: Easy | **Time**: 20-25 minutes

Ingredients Needed:
- Olive oil - divided (3 = 2 +1 tbsp.)
- Unsalted butter (1 tbsp.)
- Peeled deveined shrimp (12 raw jumbo - approx. 26-30 per lb.)
- Tilapia/another white fish (4 filets)
- Onion (1 medium - finely minced
- Garlic (1 clove)
- Heavy cream (.5 cup)
- Dry white wine (.5 cup)
- Dried thyme (.5 tsp.)
- Salt and pepper (as desired)
- Optional: Minced parsley (2 tbsp.)

Preparation Guidelines:
1. Set the oven at 150° Fahrenheit.
2. Warm a skillet and melt two tablespoons of oil with the butter (med-high temperature setting).
3. Peel and devein the shrimp. Sauté them for about two minutes per side or until almost thoroughly cooked. Remove to an oven-safe dish and set it to the side for now.
4. Next, fry the fish fillets in the same skillet until almost done (2-3 min. per side). Add the shrimp and fish in a container - covered loosely with foil and place them in the oven to keep warm.

5. Prepare the sauté pan with the rest of the oil (1 tbsp.). Mince and add the garlic and shallot. Sauté until they're softened slightly.

6. Pour in the wine and boil it using the high-temperature setting until reduced by half (1-2 min.). Stir in the cream, salt, thyme, and pepper. Adjust the temperature setting to low and simmer another minute - not boiling.

7. Divide the shrimp and fish into serving plates. Serve them with the creamy sauce and freshly minced parsley as desired.

8. Notes*** You can substitute with flounder, red snapper, or ocean perch.

☐

Manicotti

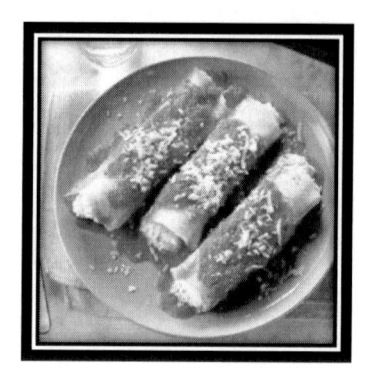

Servings: 6 | **Difficulty**: Easy | **Time**: 20-25 minutes

Ingredients Needed:
- Manicotti pasta (1 box - 8 oz./more if desired)
- Ricotta cheese (15 oz.)
- Eggs (2 - lightly beaten)
- Sugar (1 tsp.)
- Pepper & salt (1 tsp. each)
- Mozzarella cheese - shredded & divided (2 + 0.5 cups)
- Grated parmesan cheese (.5 cups)
- Spaghetti sauce (24 oz. jar)
- Also Needed: 9 by 13-inch pan

Preparation Guidelines:
1. Prepare the manicotti according to the directions on the back of the package (approx. 10 min.).
2. While it's cooking, toss all the fixings in a mixing container except the extra ½ cup of mozzarella cheese and the sauce.
3. Rinse and drain the manicotti noodles and fill each one using spoonfuls of the filling.
4. Layer the filled shells into the pan. Add the sauce all over the shells and top it off using the rest of the mozzarella cheese and a dusting of grated parmesan cheese, if desired.
5. Bake it at 350° Fahrenheit for about half an hour. □

Ravioli di Portobello

Servings: 6/15 - 20 dumplings | **Difficulty**: Difficult | **Time**: 1.5 hours

Ingredients Needed:
The Filling:
- Portobello mushrooms (1 lb.)
- Onion (1)
- Butter (.25 cup)
- Black pepper and salt (to your liking)
- Dumpling Wrappers:
- Cake flour (1.5 cups)
- Eggs (2)
- Salt (.5 tbsp.)
- Baking powder (2 tbsp.)

Sun-Dried Sauce:
- **White sauce** (2 cups **)
- Sun-dried tomatoes - chopped (2-3)
- Smoked Gouda cheese (8 oz.)

**White Sauce:
- ✓ Milk (2 cups)
- ✓ Flour (.25 cup)
- ✓ Butter (.25 cup)

Preparation Guidelines:
1. Prepare the filling. Peel the onion and dice it with the mushrooms.
2. Use a skillet to melt butter. Sauté the onion until it's transparent (5 min.).
3. Fold in the mushrooms and sauté them using the high-temperature setting until the liquid is evaporated (5 min.). Lower the setting and sauté an additional four to five minutes.
4. Remove the pan to a cool burner to chill for a few minutes. Put the mixture inside the dough.
5. Gently arrange the dumplings into boiling water to cook (20 min.).
6. Melt the rest of the butter and mix in with the ravioli to serve.
7. Prepare the wrappers. Thoroughly mix each of the fixings. Roll the dough on a flat surface until it's about ¼-inch thick (making circles).
8. Spread some water on the edges and load them with mushroom mixture. Fold in half and gently squeeze to create the dumpling. Continue the process, boiling for two minutes, or until they float to the top.
9. Prepare the sauce. Prepare a saucepan using the medium temperature setting, add the butter, whisk in the flour, and simmer for about three minutes. Stir in the milk until thickened (2 min.).
10. Mix in the chopped sun-dried tomatoes and gouda cheese using the med-low temperature setting until the cheese is melted.
11. Pour the delicious sauce over the dumplings with a portion of chopped tomatoes and onions.

Steak Gorgonzola-Alfredo

Servings: 2 | **Difficulty**: Medium | **Time**: varies according to steak doneness

Ingredients Needed:
- Steak - New York strip - sirloin or ribeye (12 oz.)
- **Black pepper & salt*** (as)
- Vegetable oil (2 tsp. desired)
- Pasta (8 oz.)
- Butter (.25 lb.)
- Heavy cream (2 cups)
- Parmesan cheese - freshly grated (.75 cup)
- Garlic powder (1 tsp.)

*Optional: Black pepper and salt
- ✓ **Sun-dried tomatoes in oil (1 oz. - chopped)**
- ✓ **Rinsed baby spinach (2 oz.)**
- ✓ **Gorgonzola cheese (2 oz.)**
- ✓ **Balsamic Glaze:**
- ✓ **Balsamic vinegar (4 oz.)**

Preparation Guidelines:
1. Season the steak using the salt and pepper. Pour two teaspoons of oil into a hot skillet and prepare the steak as you like it. Set it aside a few minutes to rest.
2. Prepare the pasta as directed on the package (8-12 min.).
3. Use the medium temperature setting to make the Alfredo sauce. Measure and combine the heavy cream and butter into a medium pot. Warm the butter and cream using the medium-temperature setting until they just begin to bubble.

4. Stir in the parmesan cheese and garlic powder until the cheese melts. Adjust the heat setting to low, and simmer until the sauce is reduced and thickened.
5. Scoop the pasta on the plate, add the rinsed spinach, and toss.
6. Pour the Alfredo sauce into the container, and place it on a serving plate with the steak portions over the pasta.
7. Top with the gorgonzola and tomatoes. Brown under the broiler until it's ready to your liking.
8. Prepare the glaze. Pour balsamic vinegar into a saucepan and warm it using the med-high temperature setting until the vinegar reduces in half.
9. Drizzle glaze over the steak just before serving.

Sides

Lasagna Dip & Pasta Chips

Servings: 8 | **Difficulty**: Medium | **Time**: 1 hour 10 minutes

Ingredients Needed:

The Chips:
- Lasagna noodles (16 oz.)

To Fry: Vegetable oil
- Garlic salt (.5 tsp.)

The Dip:
- Marinara sauce (24 oz.)
- Ground beef (4 oz.)
- Ground Italian sausage (8 oz.)
- Italian seasoning (.5 tsp.)
- Ricotta cheese (16 oz.)
- Mozzarella cheese - shredded (2 cups)
- Shredded parmesan cheese (.25 cup)

Preparation Guidelines:
1. Prepare a large dutch oven or similar pot of salted boiling water, and simmer the flat lasagna noodles until al dente. Pour them into a colander to drain - using caution not to tear the noodles.
2. While the noodles are cooking, warm the oil (360° Fahrenheit approx.).
3. Gentry pat-dry the noodles using a paper towel.
4. Work in small batches until all of the noodles are cooked. Arrange several of the lasagna noodles into the hot oil and fry until crispy and golden brown . Place the noodles in a wire rack to cool and sprinkle them using the garlic salt.
5. Prepare the dip. Set the oven at 375° Fahrenheit.
6. Warm a large saucepan using the medium-temperature setting and cook the sausage and the ground beef until the meat has browned. Break up the meat into small pieces while cooking. Drain the meat, and add it back into the saucepan.
7. Pour in the marinara sauce and Italian seasoning to the meats. Simmer until heated or for about ten minutes.
8. Use a one-quart, deep casserole dish or a 12-inch iron skillet to make the dip. Pour half of the sauce into the pan. Spread all of the ricotta cheese in the bottom in the dish.
9. Add half of the mozzarella and the rest of the sauce. Top with rest of the cheese, and parmesan.
10. Cook it for about 25 minutes to warm the dip, and if desired - set the oven to broil and brown the cheese.
11. Serve the dip with the pasta chips.

Parmesan Roasted Asparagus

Servings: 2-4 | **Difficulty**: Easy | **Time**: 45-50 minutes

Ingredients Needed:
- Fresh asparagus (1 lb.)
- Vegetable oil (2 tbsp.)
- Balsamic vinegar (1 cup)
- Salt (1 tsp.)
- Heavy cream (.5 cup)
- For the Sauce: Grated parmesan cheese (2 tbsp.)

The Garnish:
- Parmesan cheese (1 tbsp.)
- Optional: 1 lemon
- Freshly chopped tomatoes - if desired (2 tsp.)

Preparation Guidelines:
1. Prepare balsamic vinegar reduction by adding one cup of balsamic vinegar to a small pot. Adjust the temperature setting to high until the mixture boils, then lower the temp and simmer for 20 minutes. The reduction should yield ½ cup of vinegar. Store the mixture in an airtight container.
2. Discard about one inch of the asparagus' end. Place them on a sheet pan and drizzle with oil and a dusting of salt.
3. Roast the asparagus using the medium-temperature setting on a grill as you rotate the veggie (10 min. approx. according to its thickness). Remove them from the grill and

squeeze half of a lemon over the asparagus. (Olive Garden omits this step, but it is delicious.)

4. Prepare pot/skillet using the low setting. Make the parmesan sauce by adding the heavy cream and two tablespoons of grated parmesan cheese. Simmer on low for about 10 to 12 minutes until it's reduced by about 20% in volume.)

5. Serve the asparagus on a plate with a drizzle of balsamic vinegar.

6. Garnish the asparagus with one tablespoon of parmesan cheese and sauce. Garnish with freshly chopped tomatoes if desired.

Dessert
Apple Carmelina

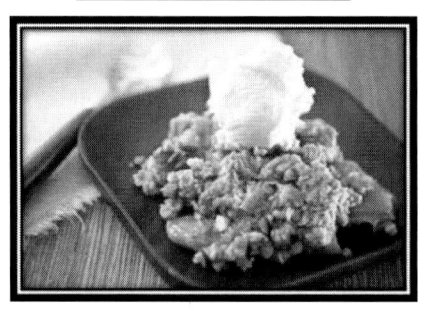

Servings: 4 | **Difficulty**: Easy | **Time**: 45 minutes

Ingredients Needed (in order as used):
- Flour (.75 cup)
- Softened butter (5 tbsp.)
- Sugar (.25 cup)
- Brown sugar (.5 cup)
- Salt (.25 tsp.)
- Sliced apples - drained (2 cans - 20 oz. each)
- Sugar (.5 cup)
- Apple pie spice (.5 tsp.)
- Brown sugar (.25 cup)
- Flour (.25 cup)
- Salt (.25 cup)
- Also Needed: 8 by 8-inch baking dish

Preparation Guidelines:
1. Warm the oven at 350° Fahrenheit.
2. Drain and slice the apples. Combine them with ½ cup of sugar, ¼ cup brown sugar, the pie spice, flour, and salt. Pour it into the lightly buttered baking dish.
3. Mix the topping fixings (sugars, flour, and salt). Mix in the softened butter until it resembles a coarse meal.
4. Drizzle the mixture over the apples and bake for 30-35 minutes. Garnish it with a drizzle of caramel sauce and scoop of vanilla ice cream (if desired).

Beverages

Berry Sangria

Servings: 8 | **Difficulty**: Very Easy | **Time**: 2 hours 5 minutes

Ingredients Needed:
- Red wine - ex. Merlot (750 ml)
- Cran-raspberry juice (2 cups)
- Simple sugar syrup (.25 cup)
- Fresh berries - ex. strawberries/blueberries/blackberries

Preparation Guidelines:
1. Add the wine, juice, and syrup in a large container. Stir and set it aside for about two hours before serving.
2. Serve the delicious drink with ice as desired, the fresh fruit, sangria, and a garnish of strawberries.
☐

<u>Watermelon Moscato Sangria</u>

Servings: 6 | **Difficulty**: Super-Easy | **Time**: 5-8 minutes

Ingredients Needed:
- Ginger ale (6 oz.)
- Moscato (750 ml.)
- Monin Watermelon Syrup (6 oz.)
- Ice (4 cups)
- Strawberries (.75 cup)
- Orange (1)
- Optional: Watermelon

Preparation Guidelines:
1. Rinse and slice the fruit into small pieces.
2. Add the fixings to a pitcher (Moscato, ginger ale & syrup).
3. Stir and add the ice.
4. Lastly, add the fruit with watermelon slices as desired.

Chapter 2: Carrabba's Italian Grill

Brunch Options

Chicken Bryan

Servings: 2 | **Difficulty**: Easy | **Time**: 30 minutes

Ingredients Needed:
- Olive oil (as needed)
- Chicken breasts (2)
- Black pepper & kosher salt (as desired)
- Goat cheese (4 oz.)
- Sun-dried tomatoes (6)
- Fresh basil (2-4 tbsp.)
- Garlic (4 tsp.)
- Onions (4 tsp.)
- Butter - divided (8 tbsp.)
- White wine (.5 cup)
- Fresh lemon juice (4 tbsp.)

Preparation Guidelines:
1. Remove all skin and bones from the chicken.
2. Chop the basil and tomatoes, and set aside for now.
3. Use olive oil to brush both sides of the chicken, dusting it with pepper and salt.
4. Arrange it on the grill and cook the chicken until done (internal temp of 165° Fahrenheit) - prepare lemon butter sauce while the chicken is grilling.
5. Dice and sauté the garlic and onions in two tablespoons of butter until softened. Mix in the wine and lemon juice.

Adjust the temperature setting to med-low and simmer ten more minutes to reduce.

6. Add the rest of the butter (6 tbsp.), a little at a time, until it melts. Fold in the chopped sun-dried tomatoes and basil, and simmer until warm.

7. Top the chicken breasts with two ounces each of the goat cheese until it's softened.

8. Serve with a spoonful of the lemon butter sauce over the delicious chicken breasts.

Lentil & Sausage Soup

Servings: 8 | **Difficulty**: Easy | **Time**: 1 hour 15 minutes

Ingredients Needed:
- Onion (1 cup)
- Carrot (.5 cup)
- Celery (.5 cup)
- Garlic (3 cloves)
- Salt (.5 tsp.)
- Butter/olive oil (2 tbsp.)
- Italian sausage (1 lb.)
- Low-sodium chicken broth (48 oz.)
- Italian seasoning (1.5 tsp.)
- Diced tomatoes (14.5 oz. can)
- Brown lentils (1 cup)

Preparation Guidelines:
1. Dice the garlic, celery, carrot, and onion.
2. Prepare a large soup pot and toss in the veggies with the butter.
3. Sauté the onions until they're translucent and mix in the sausage, cooking until browned.
4. Drain excess oil and add the diced tomatoes, lentils, tomatoes, broth, and Italian seasoning.
5. Place a lid on the pot and simmer for about one hour. Add water as needed.
6. Serve when it's as desired.

Sicilian Chicken Soup

Servings: 10 | **Difficulty**: Easy | **Time**: 2 hours 55 minutes

Ingredients Needed:
- Whole chicken (4-5 lb.)
- Russet/baking potatoes (2 medium)
- Yellow onion (1)
- Celery (4 ribs)
- Carrots (3) or Mini carrots (12)
- Red bell peppers (2)
- Diced tomatoes (14.5 oz. can)
- Fresh flat-leaf Italian parsley (.5 cup)
- Garlic cloves (5 minced)
- Black pepper & kosher salt (as desired)
- Ditalini pasta (.5 lb.)

Preparation Guidelines:

1. Remove the giblets from the chicken. Finely chop the onions, celery, peppers, and carrots. Peel and dice the potatoes (½-inch chunks).
2. Prepare a soup pot with the peppers, celery, carrots, onion potatoes, the whole chicken, and diced tomatoes (with juices). Add cold water to cover the fixings by about one inch. Set the temperature on high until boiling. Stir in the salt (1 tbsp.), pepper, parsley, and garlic.
3. Adjust the setting to med-low and place a lid on the pot (slightly ajar). Simmer for two hours until the chicken falls from the bone.
4. Remove the chicken and place it in a 'holding' container to cool for half an hour until it's easily handled. Shred the meat.
5. Lower the soup temperature to low and simmer.
6. Prepare the pasta as directed per the package instructions. Drain in a colander and set aside for now.
7. Mash the soup several times using a potato masher (2-3 times).
8. Add the chicken back into the pot and serve with the noodles to the side or any way you like them.

☐

Dinner Options
Delicious Meatballs

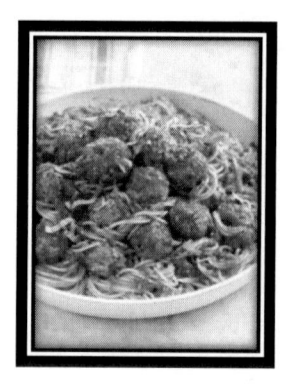

Servings: 4 | **Difficulty**: Easy| **Time**: 35-40 minutes

Ingredients Needed:
- Ground meat: 8 oz. each:
✓ Beef
✓ Pork
✓ Veal

- Whisked eggs (2)
- Grated parmesan cheese (.25 cup)
- Garlic (4 cloves)
- Breadcrumbs (1/3 cup)
- Fresh parsley (.25 cup)
- Pepper and salt (to your liking)
- Olive oil (1/3 to 1 cup)

Preparation Guidelines:
1. Set the oven temperature at 375° Fahrenheit.
2. Finely chop and sauté the garlic. Finely chop the parsley.
3. Combine all of the fixings except for the oil in a medium mixing container.
4. Warm the oil in a large-sized skillet using the med-high temperature setting.
5. Roll the mixture into 1.5-inch balls and cook until they're browned evenly - not thoroughly cooked.
6. Transfer them to a paper towel-lined platter using a slotted spoon.
7. Put the meatballs in a baking pan to bake for 20-25 minutes until they are thoroughly cooked.
8. Add sauce as desired and continue cooking until it's heated and ready to serve.
☐

Lasagna

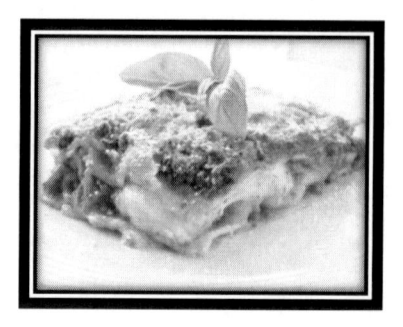

Servings: 12 | **Difficulty**: Easy | **Time**: 2 hours 40 minutes

Ingredients Needed:
- Sweet Italian sausage (1 lb.)
- Ground beef (.75 lb.)
- Onion (.5 cup)
- Garlic (2 cloves)
- Crushed tomatoes (28 oz.)
- Tomato paste (12 oz.)
- Tomato sauce (13 oz.)
- Water (.5 cup)
- White sugar (2 tbsp.)
- Dried basil (1.5 tsp.)
- Fennel seeds (.5 tsp.)
- Italian seasoning (1 tsp.)
- Pepper (.25 tsp.)
- Salt (1 tbsp.)
- Freshly chopped parsley (4 tbsp.)
- Lasagna noodles (12)
- Egg (1)
- Ricotta cheese (16 oz.)
- Salt (.5 tsp.)
- Mozzarella cheese - sliced (.75 lb.)
- Parmesan cheese - grated (.75 cup)
- *Also Needed*: 9x13-inch baking dish

Preparation Guidelines:
1. Mince/dice the onion and garlic. Prep a large skillet using the medium temperature setting, and add them with the beef and sausage. Simmer until browned and add in the water and tomatoes (paste, crushed, and sauce). Measure and mix in the fennel, basil, sugar, salt, pepper, parsley, and Italian seasoning.
2. Place a lid on the skillet and simmer for 1.5 hours.
3. Meanwhile, prepare the noodles in a pot of salted - boiling water for about eight minutes. Drain them in a colander, rinsing with fresh water.
4. Prepare a large container with the egg, mozzarella, ricotta cheese, and salt.
5. Warm the oven at 375° Fahrenheit. Lightly grease the baking dish.
6. Pour 1.5 cups of the meat sauce into the dish and layer in the six noodles with half of the cheese mix. Cover with 1/3 of the cheese fillings.
7. Continue the layers and dust with the parmesan. Cover with a layer of foil.
8. Set the timer and bake it for 25 minutes. Discard the foil and bake it for another 25 minutes.
9. Transfer the dish to a cool space.
10. Wait ten minutes before serving.

Mussels in White Wine Sauce

Servings: 4 | **Difficulty**: Medium | **Time**: 30 minutes

Ingredients Needed - Step 1:
- Mussels (4 cups) 2 tbsp. of each:
- Olive oil
- Yellow onion
- Garlic
- Pernod (licorice-flavored liqueur from France)
- Fresh basil
- Lemon juice

Ingredients Needed-Butter Sauce-Step 2:
- Clarified butter **(2 tbsp./as needed)
- Garlic (2 tbsp.)
- Onion (2 tbsp.)
- Lemon juice (6 tbsp.)
- Dry white wine (2 tbsp.)

Preparation Guidelines:
1. Prepare the ingredients in step 1. Chop the onion, garlic, and basil.
2. Also, chop and measure the garlic and onion for the butter sauce (step 2).
3. Fill a container of cold water and soak the mussels for several minutes. Use a stiff brush to remove the fibers/beard from the shell. Rinse thoroughly with cool water.
4. Warm the oil a 10-inch skillet using the medium-temperature setting.
5. Place a lid over the pot and cook the shells (2 min.) until they start opening. Remove the top and toss in the garlic and onion (stir well).

6. Cover the skillet and simmer one more minute. Transfer the pan to a cool burner and mix in the Pernod, juice, basil, and butter sauce.
7. Place it back on the burner and cook about 30-45 seconds with the lid on the pan.
8. If you have any unopened mussels, trash them and serve the remainder in a deep dish.
9. To serve, drizzle with lemon and simmer for two to three minutes and remove from the burner. Swirl in cold butter until the sauce is creamy.
10. Toss the butter sauce ingredients.
11. Note ** Clarified Butter: Melt ½ stick of butter using the low-temperature setting. Set it aside for a few minutes until the milk solids settle to the bottom of the pan. Skim the (clarified) butter from the top and trash the rest. It's okay to do this in advance and place it in the fridge to chill.
12. Make the sauce by warming the clarified butter with the garlic and onions. Sauté them until transparent and add the juice, wine, salt, and pepper as desired.

Sauces

The Grill's Seasoning

Servings: As desired| **Difficulty**: Easy | **Time**: 5 minutes

Ingredients Needed:
- Kosher salt (.25 cup)
- Kosher salt (.25 cup)
- Crushed red pepper (.25 tsp.)
- Freshly cracked black pepper (2 tbsp.)

- 1.5 tsp. of each:
- ✓ Granulated onion
- ✓ Dry oregano
- ✓ Granulated garlic

Preparation Guidelines:
1. Combine all of the fixings in a small container with a closed lid.
2. Use as desired.
☐

Italian Butter

Servings: 8 | **Difficulty**: Super-Easy | **Time**: 10 minutes

Ingredients Needed:
- Red pepper flakes (.25 tsp.)
- Black pepper (.25 tsp.)

- Spices (1/8 tsp.):
✓ Oregano
✓ Basil
✓ Kosher salt
✓ Rosemary
✓ Garlic (2 tsp.)
✓ Olive oil (3 tbsp.)

Preparation Guidelines:
1. Prepare the mixture in a small mixing container.
2. Crush the garlic and mix it with all the dry spices.
3. Whisk in the oil and dip it using your favorite bread.

Chapter 3: Biaggi's Ristorante Italiano Restaurant

Brunch Options
__Formaggi di Capra__

Servings: 5 | **Difficulty**: Easy | **Time**: 30 minutes

Ingredients Needed:
- Goat cheese (12 oz.)
- Cream cheese (.5 cup)
- Fresh thyme (2 tsp.)
- Chives (2 tbsp.)
- Fresh parsley (2 tbsp.)
- Marinara sauce (1 cup)
- Kalamata olives (8)
- Baguette/cut on the bias (10 slices)
- Butter (4 tbsp.)
- Pureed garlic (1 tsp.)
- Parmesan cheese - grated (.25 cup)

Preparation Guidelines:
1. Warm the oven to reach 350° Fahrenheit.
2. Prep the veggies by chopping the parsley, chives, and thyme. Remove the pits from the olives.
3. Melt the butter in a small mixing container. Mix in the garlic puree.
4. Slice the bread into about ten slices.
5. Brush garlic butter over the surfaces of each slice of bread. Arrange the slices onto a baking tray to cook for five to six minutes.
6. Flip the slices and dust using parmesan cheese. Pop the tray back into the oven and bake for another three to four minutes.
7. Measure and add the cream cheese, goat cheese, thyme, parsley, and chives in a mixing bowl and blend. Empty the mixture into a baking dish to cook until the cheese is slightly brown (4-6 min.).
8. Transfer it to the countertop and pour in the marinara sauce to continue baking (2-3 min.). Transfer the baking pan to the countertop and garnish it using the olives.
9. Arrange the baking dish on a large platter and add the toasted bread slices around the tray to serve promptly.

Mushroom Chicken Alfredo

Servings: 3-4 | **Difficulty**: Easy | **Time**: 30 minutes not including cook time for the chicken)

Ingredients Needed:
- Alfredo sauce (2.5 cups)
- Chicken broth (.75 cup)
- Cooked rotisserie chicken (1.5 cups - pulled)
- Wild mushrooms, sliced (.5 cup)
- Garlic puree (.5 tsp.)
- Italian parsley - chopped (.25 tsp.)
- Walnuts - chopped (.25 cup)
- Grated parmesan cheese (.25 cup)
- Black pepper & salt (.25 tsp. each)
- Gemelli pasta (16 oz.)
- Freshly cracked black pepper (.25 tsp.)
- Fresh basil (4 sprigs)

Preparation Guidelines:
1. Pour the broth, alfredo sauce, sliced mushrooms, walnuts, garlic puree, pulled chicken, salt, pepper, and parsley in a large-sized skillet. Stir and wait for it to boil.
2. Adjust the temperature setting to low to simmer for one minute. Transfer the pan to a cool burner, cover, and set the pan aside.
3. Cook the pasta per the package instructions (approx. 8-12 min.).
4. Drain most of the water (90 percent) and pour in the sauce with the pasta. Stir it using the med-high temperature setting for one to two minutes. Remove the pan from the burner.
5. Serve it with a garnish of freshly ground pepper (in addition to step 1) and basil to serve.
☐

Ravioli Romano

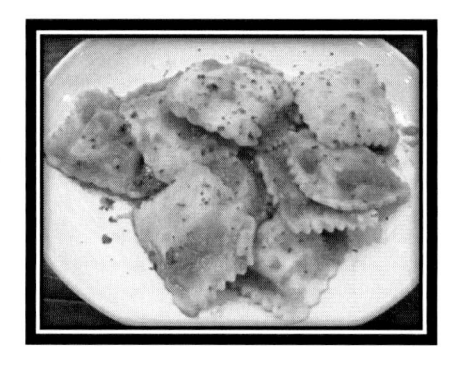

Servings: 3-4 | **Difficulty**: Easy | **Time**: 15 minutes

Ingredients Needed:
- Water (approx. 3 quarts)
- Frozen beef ravioli (16 oz.)
- Unsalted butter (.25 cup)
- Fresh sage (1 tbsp.)
- Salt & pepper (1 tsp. each)
- Parsley (1 tbsp.)
- Chicken broth (.5 cup)
- Red pasta sauce (.5 cup)
- Toasted pine nuts (.25 cup)
- Fresh spinach - julienned (.5 cup)
- Grated Asiago cheese (2 tbsp.)

Preparation Guidelines:
1. Warm a sauté pan to melt the butter using the med-high temperature setting until it resembles the shade of dark brown sugar.
2. Roughly chop the sage and parsley. Toss them into the heated pan with pepper and salt.
3. Pour in the chicken broth, red sauce, and pine nuts. Wait for the mixture to boil and remove it to a cool burner. Set it to the side for now.
4. Prepare the ravioli. Warm a large stockpot with about three quarts of water. Heat it until it is boiling using the high-temperature setting. Cook, uncovered, for four to six minutes, or until they are heated through and begin to float.
5. Drain 90 percent of the water from the pan.
6. Mix in the spinach and sauce with the ravioli. Gently toss and simmer (high setting) for 20-30 seconds.
7. Adjust the seasonings to your liking.
8. Serve the delicious ravioli with a garnish of cheese to serve.

☐

Tuscan Country Salad

Servings: 2-4 | **Difficulty**: Super-Easy | **Time**: 15 minutes

Ingredients Needed:
- Romaine lettuce (1 lb.)
- Creamy parmesan dressing (.75 cup)
- Ham (.5 cup)
- Turkey (.5 cup)
- Swiss cheese (.5 cup)
- Mozzarella cheese (.5 cup)
- Danish blue cheese (.25 cup)
- Red onions (.25 cup)
- Black olives (.5 cup)
- Plum tomatoes (.5 cup)
- Hard-boiled egg (1 sliced)
- Pepperoncini (4)
- Bacon - cooked & diced (2 tbsp.)

Preparation Guidelines:
1. Dice or chop the lettuce, onions, olives, tomatoes, egg, cheese, and meats.
2. Toss the lettuce and dressing in a large mixing container until the salad is evenly covered.
3. Fold in and toss the ham, turkey, cheeses, onions, olives, and tomatoes.
4. Slice and add in the hard-boiled egg on top of the salad. Sprinkle bacon on top of the mixture and serve.
5. Note: The time does not count cooking the bacon or egg.

Dinner Options
<u>Garmugia Soup</u>

Servings: 6 | Difficulty: Easy | Time: 1 hour

Ingredients Needed:
- Olive oil (2 tbsp.)
- Garlic cloves (4)
- Spanish onions (.5 cup)
- Celery (.5 cup)
- Leeks (.5 cup)
- Asparagus (.5 cup)
- Broccoli florets (.5 cup)
- Green beans (.5 cup)
- Escarole (.5 cup)
- Fresh peas (.5 cup)
- Savoy cabbage (.5 cup)
- Zucchini (.5 cup)
- Fresh spinach (.25 cup)
- Water (8 cups)
- Salt and black pepper (.5 tbsp.)

Preparation Guidelines:
1. Chop or dice the veggies for the soup.
2. Warm the olive oil in a two-gallon stockpot. Once it's hot, toss in the garlic and onions to sauté them until the onions are tender (3-4 min.).
3. Add the rest of the fixings and wait for it to boil. Adjust the temperature setting to simmer for about half an hour.
4. Ladle the hot soup into individual serving bowls and garnish with a splash of oil and freshly ground black pepper.

Pork Chops Milanese

Servings: 2 | **Difficulty**: Easy | **Time**: 1 hour

Ingredients Needed:
- Milk (1.5 cups)
- Flour (1 cup)
- Eggs (2)
- Water (2 tbsp.)
- Vegetable oil (.75 cup)
- Pork chops (2 @ 10 oz. each)
- Breadcrumbs (1 cup)
- Lemon (1 - zested @ 1 tsp. & juice @ 2 tbsp.)
- Black pepper and salt (1 dash each)
- Olive oil (6 tbsp.)
- Arugula (.5 cup)
- Capers (2 tbsp.)
- Cherry tomatoes (6)
- Red onion (2 tbsp. - julienned)
- Asiago cheese (.25 cup)

Preparation Guidelines:
1. Marinate the pork chops in a large mixing container by adding the milk over them. Place a top/foil on the container and pop it into the fridge for one hour.
2. At that time, transfer the chops from the marinade and dip them into the flour. Use a shallow container and whisk the water with the eggs. Plunge the floured chops in the egg wash. Lastly, dip them in breadcrumbs until they are thoroughly covered.
3. Prepare a large skillet using the medium setting to heat the oil. Once the pan starts to smoke, promptly add the prepared chops. Fry them for approximately two minutes per side.
4. Toss the arugula, capers, tomatoes, and red onions in a small mixing container.
5. In another container, whisk the lemon juice, zested lemon, pepper, salt, and oil until thoroughly mixed.

6. Dress and toss the salad with dressing. Serve it alongside the pork chops on the plate with a portion of shaved cheese.

Sauce

Alfredo Sauce

Servings: 8/Yields 1 quart | **Difficulty**: Easy | **Time**: 15 minutes

Ingredients Needed:
- Butter (⅛ cup)
- Pureed garlic (5 tbsp.)
- Finely diced yellow onion (.25 cup)
- Milk (2.5 cups)
- Heavy cream (1 cup)
- Ground nutmeg (1 dash)
- Black pepper (.25 tsp.)
- Salt (.75 tsp.)
- Water (3 tbsp.)
- Parmesan cheese (⅜ cup)

Preparation Guidelines:
1. Melt butter in a saucepan using the medium temperature setting. Pour in the pureed garlic and diced onions. Sauté them for five minutes until the onions are tender.
2. Whisk in the cream, milk, nutmeg, salt, and pepper.
3. Dissolve the cornstarch in water, mixing well so that there are no lumps. Slowly add the cornstarch mixture (just as the sauce comes to a boil) and whisk well.
4. Remove the pan to a cool burner to stir in the cheeses for three or more minutes until the sauce is very smooth.
5. Note: You may use a regular blender if desired, but use caution with the hot sauce. Puree one to two cups at a time. The use of a blender is optional.
6. Season the sauce to your liking. Keep it warm or cool, and store it in the fridge until needed.

Side Dish

Biscotti di Prato

Servings: 2 dozen | **Difficulty**: Easy | **Time**: 30-35 minutes

Ingredients Needed:
- Granulated sugar (.75 cup)
- Unsalted butter - softened (.5 cup)
- Eggs (2 large)
- Almond extract (.25 tsp.)
- Baking powder (1.5 tsp.)
- Salt (.25 tsp.)
- Cinnamon (.25 tsp.)
- A-P flour (2.5 cups)
- Almonds - sliced (1 cup)

Preparation Guidelines:
1. Set the oven temperature at 350° Fahrenheit. Prepare a baking tray with a layer of parchment baking paper. Whisk the sugar and butter in a large mixing container.
2. Slowly, mix in the eggs. Stir well and mix in the cinnamon, salt, baking powder, and almond extract - until just blended. Gradually fold in the flour (if using a mixer - use the low-speed setting).
3. Fold in the almonds, and combine about half of a minute. Form the dough into a 12 by 3-inch log. Arrange it on the baking sheet.
4. Bake until lightly golden (40 min.). Cool for half an hour. Cut diagonally into ¾-inch slices. Adjust the temperature setting to 300° Fahrenheit. Arrange the slices (cut side down).
5. Set a timer to bake for 15-20 minutes.
6. Switch the pan to the countertop and cool the biscotti for about an hour

Dessert

Biaggi's Ristorante Italiano Barolo Zabaione

Servings: 6 | **Difficulty**: Medium | **Time**: 15 minutes

Ingredients Needed:
- Egg yolks (6)
- Granulated sugar (.5 cup)
- Heavy cream (1 cup)
- Barolo wine (.75 cup)
- Blueberries (.5 cup)
- Freshly pinched mint (6 sprigs)

Preparation Guidelines:
1. Prepare a double boiler halfway with water and wait for it to boil using the med-high temperature setting.
2. Transfer the pan from the burner, and add and whisk the fixings into the top of the boiler (eggs, sugar, and half of the Barolo wine). Simmer for five minutes, stirring continuously.
3. Pour in the rest of the wine and whisk until it's thickened. Transfer the pan to an ice bath to cool.
4. Prepare a large mixing container and whisk the heavy cream until it forms firm peaks. Combine and mix the fixings.
5. Portion the tasty mixture into small serving dishes or shot glasses. Toss in a few blueberries and sprigs of mint to serve.

Chapter 4: Fazoli's Favorites

If you are looking for a super-easy recipe for breadsticks; you are in the right place:

Brunch Options
Grilled Chicken Panini

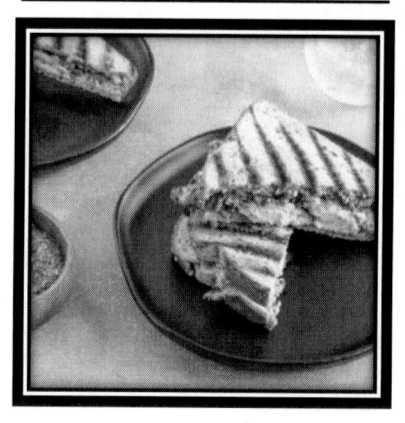

Servings: 1 | **Difficulty**: Easy | **Time**: 10-15 minutes

Ingredients Needed:
- Focaccia bread (1 grilled)
- Lite Italian dressing - your preference (1 oz.)
- Grilled chicken breast - hot (1 whole)
- Oregano (2 shakes)
- Provolone cheese (.5 oz.)
- Romaine lettuce (1 head)
- Tomato (2 slices)

Preparation Guidelines:
1. Slice the loaf of focaccia into lengthwise pieces. Cover each side using the Italian dressing.
2. Grill the chicken and slice it thinly to your liking (time not allotted in counts) or purchase it pre-cut and cooked.
3. Arrange the chicken onto the focaccia, adding the oregano, provolone, lettuce, and tomato.
☐

Stuffed Seafood Shells

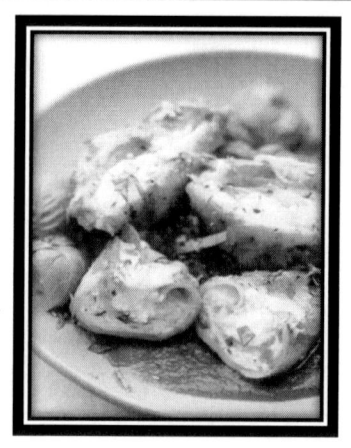

Servings: 4 | **Difficulty**: Easy | **Time**: 40 minutes

Ingredients Needed:
- Ricotta cheese (8 oz.)
- Egg (1 beaten)
- Mozzarella cheese (.5 cup)
- Small shrimp (1 small can or .5 cup)
- Lobster (8 oz.)
- Garlic salt (1 pinch)
- Alfredo sauce (1 jar commercial)
- Large stuffing shells (12 oz. pkg.)
- Spaghetti (1 lb.)
- Tomato sauce (as desired)
- **Also Needed**: 8-inch square baking pan

Preparation Guidelines:
1. Set the oven at 350° Fahrenheit.
2. Steam and chop the shrimp. Prepare the shells and spaghetti per the package instructions. When ready, mix the egg with the ricotta cheese. Stir in the lobster, shrimp, mozzarella cheese, and garlic salt. Prepare the shells with the mixture.
3. Pour a little sauce (as you like it) into the baking pan and add the shells, pouring additional sauce over the shells.
4. Place a foil/lid layer on the pan and bake until hot (20-25 min.).
5. Serve the delicious meal over spaghetti with a portion of tomato sauce.

Dinner Options
Baked Beef & Spaghetti

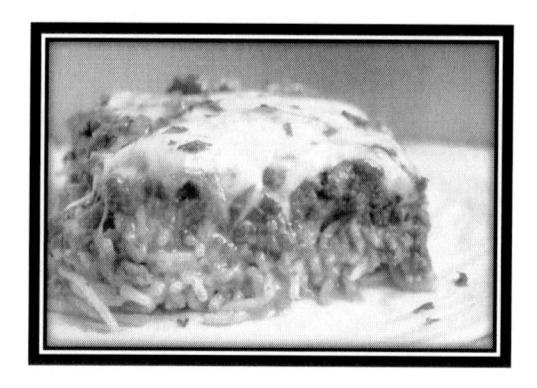

Servings: 4-6 | Difficulty: Easy | Time: 1.25 to 1.5 hours

Ingredients Needed:
- Spaghetti (16 oz. pkg.)
- Ground beef (1 lb.)
- Onion (1 medium)
- Meatless spaghetti sauce (24 oz. jar)
- Seasoned salt (.5 tsp.)
- Eggs (2)
- Parmesan cheese - grated (1/3 cup)
- Butter - melted (5 tbsp.)
- Shredded mozzarella cheese (2 cups/16 oz.)
- *Also Needed*: 1 greased 3-quart baking dish

Preparation Guidelines:
1. Cook spaghetti according to package instructions (8-12 min.).
2. Warm the oven at 350° Fahrenheit.
3. Dice the onion and toss it into a large skillet and sauté them using the medium temperature setting until the meat is no longer pink. Drain the juices from the skillet, and add the seasoned salt and spaghetti sauce. Set the pan to the side.
4. Combine the butter with the parmesan and the whisked eggs.
5. Drain and mix in the spaghetti, tossing to coat.
6. Pour about ½ of the spaghetti mixture into the prepared baking dish. Top with half of the meat sauce and a portion of mozzarella. Duplicate the layers.
7. Place a lid or layer of foil over the dish and bake it for 40 minutes.
8. Discard the lid/foil and continue baking until the cheese is melted (20-25 min.).
☐

Baked Garlic Chicken Spaghetti

Servings: 8-12 | **Difficulty**: Easy |
Time: 50-55 minutes

Ingredients Needed:
- Olive oil - divided (2 tbsp.)
- Biscuit mix (.5 cup)
- Grated parmesan cheese (2 tbsp.)
- Basil (1 tsp.)
- Garlic powder (.5 tsp.)
- Pepper (.25 tsp.)
- Oregano (1 tsp.)
- Chicken breast (4 halves - boneless)
- Tomato sauce (1 quart)
- Spaghetti sauce (28 oz. can)
- Garlic (3-5 minced cloves)
- Shredded mozzarella cheese - divided (3 cups)
- Linguine - cooked & drained (12 oz. pkg.)
- Parmesan cheese (.5 cup - set aside for later)
- *Also Needed*: 13x9-inch pan and skillet

Preparation Guidelines:
1. Warm a skillet using the med-high temperature setting and warm the oven at 350° Fahrenheit. Grease the pan with one tablespoon of oil.
2. Mix the biscuit mix, parmesan, oregano, basil, garlic, and pepper in a small mixing container.
3. Pull "tenders" from the breast halves and dip them into the biscuit mixture.
4. Add the remainder of the oil to the hot pan and brown the chicken pieces, flipping them to ensure they are evenly browned. Remove the pan to a cold burner.
5. Meanwhile, whisk the spaghetti sauce with the tomato, mix in the garlic, adding additional spices as desired.ish.

6. Spread a layer (1/3) of cooked pasta over the pan. Dust it using about 1/4 of the mozzarella.
7. Spread about a cup of the sauce over this. Duplicate the layers two times (reserving about one cup of the cheese).
8. Layer the pieces of chicken over the last layer of pasta-cheese-sauce. Add the remainder of the sauce over the meat, and dust on the rest of the mozzarella.
9. Bake in the heated oven to cook for about half an hour.
10. For the final phase, dust the dish with the remainder of the parmesan and bake for ten additional minutes.
11. Serve when it's golden brown.

Side Dish
Delicious Breadsticks

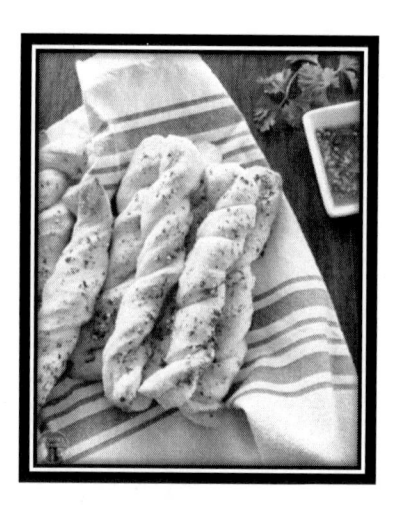

Servings: 6 | **Difficulty**: Super-Easy | **Time**: 10 minutes

Ingredients Needed:
- Plain breadsticks (10.5 oz. frozen pkg.)
- Margarine (1 cup)
- Kosher salt (up to 3 tbsp.)

Preparation Guidelines:
1. Arrange the breadsticks in a baking tray.
2. In a mixing container, combine the margarine and salt. Stir and brush it over the breadsticks.
3. Bake at 400° Fahrenheit until they're nicely browned.

Chapter 5: Original Sicilian Pasta Co.

Brunch Option
Calabrese

Servings: 2 | **Difficulty**: Easy | **Time**: 20 minutes

Ingredients Needed:
- Olive oil (.25 cup)
- Capers (.5 tbsp.)
- Garlic (1 tsp.)
- Butterflied shrimp (5)
- White wine (2 oz.)
- Pepper and salt (1 pinch)
- Blanched broccoli (4 florets)
- Basil leaves (2 large)
- Sun-dried tomatoes (2 large)
- Clam broth (2 oz.)
- Butter (1 tbsp.)
- Cooked linguine (10 oz. pkg.)

Preparation Guidelines:
1. Mince the garlic and butterfly the shrimp. Slice the basil leaves and dried tomatoes. Toss all of the fixings into a skillet and sauté them until the shrimp are done.
2. Pour in the cooked linguine and toss (Cook it as directed on the package.).
3. Add the shrimp to a platter with the broccoli and pasta in the center with a freshly minced batch of basil and parsley.

Dinner Options
Calamari Bolognese

Servings: 10 | **Difficulty**: Easy | **Time**: 25-30 minutes

Ingredients Needed:
- Squid (4 lb.)
- Onions (2 cups)
- Olive oil (.5 cup)
- Celery (2 cups)
- Carrots (2 cups)
- Garlic (.5 cup)
- Saffron threads (.5 tsp.)
- Vermouth (1 cup)
- Tomato sauce (6 cups)
- Pepper & salt (as desired)
- Deep-fried breaded squid (.5 lb.)
- Pasta ribbons - al dente (4 lb.)

Preparation Guidelines:
1. First, clean the squid and prepare it in batches. Coarsely chop it using a food processor and chill it in the refrigerator.
2. Dice and sauté the onions in oil until 'just' wilted. Mince/dice the garlic, celery, and carrots. Add them to the mixture with the saffron to sauté about one to two minutes. Add the squid, cooking fast to evaporate the liquids.
3. Pour in the vermouth and simmer/reduce until almost dry. Stir in the seasonings and tomato sauce.
4. If you want to break it into individual servings, warm two cups of sauce with eight ounces of pasta. Toss and garnish with the fried tentacles.
5. It's even tastier if stored in the fridge overnight.
6. When serving or reheating, mix the salad - placing the pepper on top with a portion of the cheese.

Party Time Sicilian Pasta Shrimp Alfredo

Servings: 24 | **Difficulty**: Easy | **Time**: 15-20 minutes

Ingredients Needed:
- Olive oil (1.5 cups)
- Shrimp (6 lb.)
- Mushrooms (36 oz)
- Garlic (6 oz.)
- Green onions (12 oz.)
- Heavy cream (6 quarts)
- Tomatoes (12 oz.)
- Grated parmesan cheese (1.5 lb.)
- Fettuccine - cooked as directed on package (9 lb.)

Preparation Guidelines:
1. Prepare a skillet and warm the oil.
2. Peel, devein, and toss in the shrimp with the sliced mushrooms, and cook for two minutes.
3. Chop and add in the garlic and scallions, cooking an additional minute (removing the shrimp when ready).
4. Pour in the cream, and simmer to reduce the liquid for five minutes.
5. Add the tomatoes and parmesan. Reduce the mixture one minute longer.
6. Toss the shrimp back into the pan with the fettuccine until heated.
7. Scoop the mixture onto the pasta plate, adding the shrimp last using a bit of basil.

Sides

Party-Time Bruschetta Spread

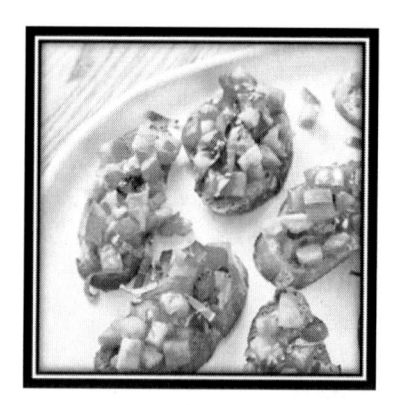

Servings: 48 | **Difficulty**: Super Easy | **Time**: 25 minutes

Ingredients Needed:
- Roasted red bell peppers (12)
- Kalamata olives (2 cups)
- Olive oil (4 tbsp.)
- Black pepper (as desired)

- *Optional Ingredients*:
- Freshly chopped rosemary
- Crushed garlic

Preparation Guidelines:
1. Prepare the bell peppers (roast, peel, deseed, and chop), and combine with the pitted and chopped olives, pepper, and oil in a mixing container.
2. Stir and let them marinate for about 15 minutes for the flavors to mix.
3. Optional Steps: Mix in the extra fixings if desired. If you don't like salty olives, soak them in olive oil to remove some of the salty taste, and use the oil as salad dressing.
☐

Stuffed Portobellos

Servings: 2-4 | **Difficulty**: Easy | **Time**: 15 minutes

Ingredients Needed:
- Portobello mushrooms (8 medium)
- Shrimp (8 oz.)
- Mushrooms (1 cup)
- Garlic powder (a pinch or 2/as desired)
- Onions (.5 cup)
- Butter (3 oz.)
- Olive oil (1 oz.)
- Garlic (1 tbsp.)
- Eggs (2 medium)
- Lobster Base (2 tbsp.)
- Breadcrumbs (2 cups)
- Parsley (1 tbsp.)
- Black pepper (1 tsp.)
- White wine (2 oz.)
- Shredded crabmeat (12 oz.)
- Mozzarella cheese - shredded (8 oz.)

Preparation Guidelines:
1. Clean and brush the mushrooms using oil. Grill until done (5-7 min.).
2. While they are grilling, devein, peel, and finely chop the mushrooms (1 cup), shrimp and onions.
3. Warm a skillet and add the oil and butter. Toss in the mushrooms, shrimp, and onions into the skillet to sauté until the shrimp turn pink.
4. Transfer the pan to a cool burner. Coarsely grind the pepper and add the rest of the fixings. Stir until it's firm. Add more breadcrumbs and an additional egg until the mixture is easily shaped into balls.

5. Scoop the mixture into the Portobello, covering it edge-to-edge. Dust it using shredded mozzarella and broil to your liking before serving.

Chapter 6: Pasta House Company

Brunch Options
Fettuccine Alfredo

Servings: 4 | **Difficulty**: Easy | **Time**: 15 minutes

Ingredients Needed:
- Fettuccine noodles (10 oz.)
- Half & Half (8 oz.)
- Butter (1 oz.)
- Parmigianino cheese (.25 cup - grated)

Preparation Guidelines:
1. Prepare a pot of salted water. Toss in the fettuccine to cook for about five to six minutes (¾ done) and drain them into a colander.
2. Add them back into the pot with the butter and cream.
3. Cook until they are done as desired and transfer to a cool burner. Add in the cheese and pepper and toss to serve.

Pasta Con Broccoli

Servings: 4-6 | **Difficulty**: Easy | **Time**: 40 minutes

Ingredients Needed:
- Broccoli (1 head)
- Cooked pasta shells (.5 lb.)
- Mushrooms (8 oz. can)
- Butter (1/2 stick)
- Half & Half (2 cups + a little bit of milk)
- Tomato sauce (8 oz.)
- Parmesan cheese (1 cup)

- *Optional - As Desired*:
- Garlic powder
- Black pepper & salt
- Also Needed: 9x13 baking pan

Preparation Guidelines:
1. Prepare a pot of boiling - salted water (1-inch in the bottom) and add an insert/steamer basket.
2. Rinse and trim the broccoli into florets. Toss them into the top of the boiler pan, cover, and steam until tender (3-8 min./as desired).
3. Slice and sauté the mushrooms in ½ stick of butter (5 min.).
4. Once the broccoli, noodles, and mushrooms have all been prepared, toss each of the fixings into a baking pan. Cover the pan with foil to bake in a 425° Fahrenheit oven until the sauce starts to thicken (20 min.).
5. Note: The sauce will continue to thicken after it's out of the oven.

Penne Primavera

Servings: 1-2 | **Difficulty**: Easy | **Time**: 15 minutes

Ingredients Needed:
- Olive oil (.5 oz.)
- Fresh broccoli (2 oz.)
- Zucchini (1 oz.)
- Fresh mushrooms (1 oz.)
- Spaghetti sauce (1 oz.)
- Cooked penne noodle (10 oz.)

Preparation Guidelines:
1. Slice the zucchini and mushrooms. Cook the noodles for about five minutes.
2. Blanch the broccoli for two to three minutes.
3. Pour the oil into a pot and add the butter, zucchini, and mushrooms. Sauté them for two minutes. Pour in the spaghetti sauce, broccoli, and the noodles.
4. Toss to heat for three minutes. Remove the noodles and arrange the vegetables on top with a Pof Parmigiano cheese.
☐

Dinner Options
Chicken Flamingo

Servings: 4 | **Difficulty**: Medium | **Time**: 40 minutes

Ingredients Needed:
- Butter (half of 1 stick/.25 cup)
- All-purpose flour (.25 cup)
- Chicken broth (1.25 cups)
- White wine (.5 cup)
- Lemon juice (.25 cup)
- Fresh broccoli (1.5 cups)
- Chicken breast halves (4)
- Olive oil (1.5 tbsp.)
- Italian breadcrumbs (1 cup)
- Red pepper flakes (.5 tsp.)
- Prosciutto (1 tbsp.)
- Garlic (2 tsp.)
- Mushrooms (1.5 cups)
- Provolone & mozzarella cheese (1 cup each - shredded)

Preparation Guidelines:
1. First, be sure all bones and skin are removed from the chicken. Prepare the broccoli into florets, chop/dice the garlic and prosciutto, and slice the mushrooms.
2. Prepare the sauce by melting the butter in a small saucepan using the medium temperature setting.
3. Whisk and add in the flour to make a roux. Adjust the range top setting to low and cook, often stirring until roux forms (3 min.). Set aside.

4. Combine the broth and lemon juice in a medium-sized saucepan. Once it's boiling, whisk in the roux. Transfer the pan from the burner and whisk in the wine until the sauce is smooth. Pop the container in the fridge until serving time.

5. Warm the grill or use the oven broiler. Also, set the oven at 450° Fahrenheit if you are using a grill.

6. Boil a saucepan of water to cook the broccoli, simmering until it's tender and bright green. Scoop the broccoli into ice water to cool. Dump it into a colander to drain, and pat it dry using a bunch of paper towels.

7. Flatten the chicken using a meat mallet (½ to ¾-inches). Coat the chicken with oil, dredging it into the platter of breadcrumbs.

8. Grill/broil the chicken at 450° Fahrenheit for about four minutes on each side (170° Fahrenheit -internal temp).

9. Pour the sauce into a large skillet. Fold in the red pepper flakes, garlic, and prosciutto. Once it's boiling, add in the mushrooms and broccoli. Simmer until the sauce thickens (reduced 1/3 in volume).

10. Combine the cheeses. Arrange the cooked chicken on a shallow baking pan and garnish it with ½ cup of cheese. Bake until the cheese is melted (4 min.).

11. Transfer the chicken to serving plates. Scoop the broccoli and mushrooms over the chicken using a slotted spoon. Pour in the rest of the sauce as desired and serve promptly.

☐

Chicken Ignatio

Servings: 4 | **Difficulty**: Easy|
Time: 20-25 minutes

Ingredients Needed:
- Chicken breast (1 lb.)
- Rigatoni (1 lb.)
- 1 % milk (4 cups)
- Knorr Parma Rosa Sauce Mix (4 - 1.3 oz. envelopes)
- Sweet Marsala wine (.5 cup)
- Prosciutto (.25 cup)
- Roasted red peppers (1 cup)
- Mushrooms (1 cup)
- Frozen peas (1 cup)
- Red pepper flakes (1 pinch)

Preparation Guidelines:
1. Remove the bones and skin from the chicken. Chop the peppers, mushrooms, and prosciutto.
2. Grill the chicken breasts, and slice them into thin strips. Cook the rigatoni until al dente, and drain. (These cooking times are not included in the total minutes' count.)
3. In a large pot, warm the milk (do not boil) and transfer it to a cool burner.
4. Slowly whisk in the marsala and Parma Rosa sauce mixing until smooth. Adjust the temperature setting to low and add in the red peppers, prosciutto, mushrooms, and frozen peas. Heat until hot.
5. Stir in the cooked chicken, cooked rigatoni, and red pepper flakes.
6. Readjust the temperature setting to medium and simmer until the sauce thickens (3-4 min.).
7. Serve the delicious meal when it's ready!
☐

Sides

Garlic Cheese Bread

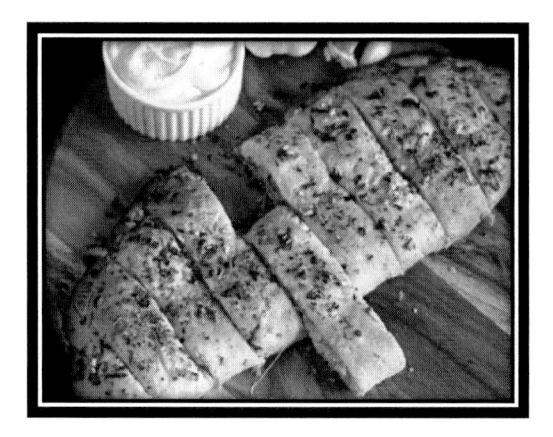

Servings: 16 | **Difficulty**: Easy | **Time**: 15 minutes

Ingredients Needed:
- French Bread (1 loaf)
- Butter (.5 cup)
- Garlic powder (1 tsp.)
- Provolone cheese (1 lb. **)

Preparation Guidelines:
1. Set the oven temperature at 375° Fahrenheit.
2. Slice the bread into slices (on the bias).
3. Melt the garlic powder and butter. Dip the bread in the butter and sprinkle with the cheese.
4. Bake until the cheese is melted.
5. Note: **You can also substitute with cheddar, mozzarella, etc.
☐

Pasta House Co. Special Salad

Servings: 4| **Difficulty**: Easy |
Time: 20-25 minutes

Ingredients Needed:
- Romaine lettuce (about 1/3 of 1 head)
- Iceberg lettuce (1 head)
- Sliced red onions (0.33 cup/as desired)
- Artichoke hearts (1 cup)
- Diced pimentos (1 cup)
- Olive oil (0.66 cup)
- Red wine vinegar (0.33 cup)
- Salt (1 tsp.)
- Freshly grated Parmigiano cheese (0.66 cup)
- Black pepper (.25 tsp.)

Preparation Guidelines:
1. Wash both types of lettuce, drain in a colander, and put it into the fridge to chill.
2. After it's thoroughly chilled, break the head of iceberg lettuce in half, pulling the heart of lettuce out of both halves and cutting them into small bite-sized chunks.
3. Rip the romaine lettuce (each leaf into three sections). Toss each type of lettuce into the salad mixing bowl.
4. Thoroughly drain and toss in the artichoke hearts.
5. Rinse, peel and slice the red onion, and drain and dice the pimentos. Toss them with the lettuce.
6. Stir in the vinegar, oil, salt, and pepper. Toss and add the Parmigiano cheese thoroughly mixing to serve.

Chapter 7: Romano's Macaroni Grill

Brunch Option
Pesto Chicken Farfalle

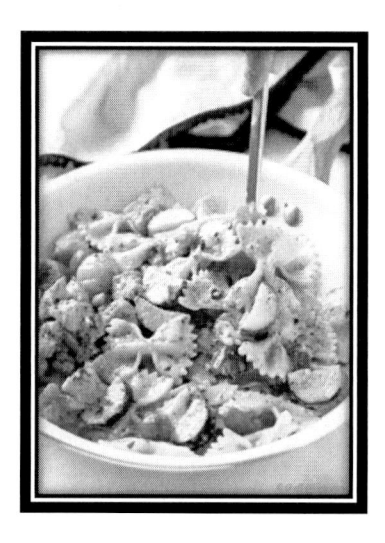

Servings: 2-3 | **Difficulty**: Easy | **Time**: 20-25 minutes

Ingredients Needed:
- Farfalle pasta (16 oz.)
- Heavy cream (1/3 cup)
- Pesto (1 cup)
- Red chili flakes (1 tsp.)
- Reserved pasta water (.5 cup)
- Chicken thighs (3)
- Black pepper and salt (as desired)
- Sun-dried tomatoes, in oil (3 tbsp.)
- Garnish: Parsley (a small handful - chopped)

Preparation Guidelines:
1. Prepare a large pot of boiling water with salt. Toss the pasta into it and cook as you like them or per the advised time on the package. Set aside ½ cup of the water before draining the pasta.
2. Remove the skin and any bones from the chicken and dust it using salt and pepper. Grill it on an indoor pan until it's to your liking (3 min. each side). Once they are slightly cooled, dice them and set aside for now.
3. Warm a large sauté pan and toss in the red chili flakes, pesto, and cream until hot (you don't want it boiling).
4. Fold in the pasta and mix in ½ cup of the chopped sundried tomatoes, diced chicken, and parsley. Adjust the seasonings as desired and serve.
☐

Dinner Options
Macaroni Grill Seafood Linguine

Servings: 6-8 | **Difficulty**: Medium | **Time**: 30 minutes

Ingredients Needed:
- Olive oil (2 tbsp.)
- Linguine (1 lb.)
- Shrimp (1 lb.)
- Bay scallop (.5 lb.)
- Garlic (3 tbsp.)
- Red pepper flakes (.75 tsp.)
- Butter (3 tbsp.)
- White wine (1.5 cups)
- Zested lemon (1 tsp.)
- Sea salt - ex. - Tuscan Seasoned (as desired)
- *Topping*: Freshly chopped parsley & black pepper

Preparation Guidelines:
1. Cook the linguine according to package directions (approx. 8-9 min.).
2. Warm the oil in a large skillet using the medium-temperature setting.
3. Peel and devein the shrimp. Mince the garlic.
4. Melt a couple of tablespoons of the butter with the oil and garlic before adding the shrimp.
5. Pour in the white wine. Once boiling, adjust the temperature setting and simmer for another three to five minutes.
6. Mix in the scallops, rest of the butter, salt, pepper, and lemon zest to simmer until it's just warmed (2 min.).
7. Drain the pasta and add it to a serving dish, add the seafood and white wine with a portion of parsley and freshly cracked black pepper.

8. Restaurant Tip - Optional Step: Add grape tomatoes and chopped arugula (as desired) to the sauce to make this a 'true' restaurant copycat recipe.

Pasta Di Mare

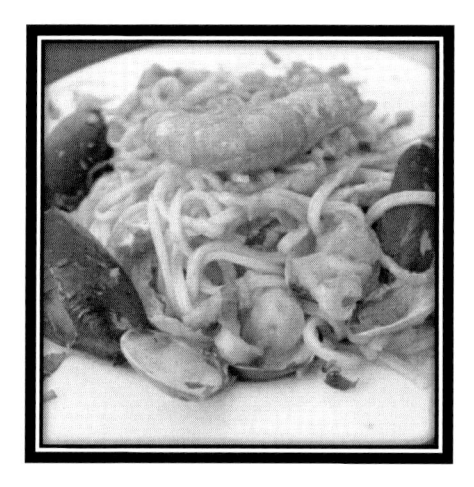

Servings: 4 | **Difficulty**: Easy | **Time**: 25-30 minutes

Ingredients Needed:
- Olive oil (1 tbsp.)
- Garlic (2 cloves)
- Dry white wine (.5 cup)
- Littleneck/manila clams (12)
- Black mussels (1 dozen)
- Shrimp (8)
- Sea scallops (4 quartered)
- Calamari - ringlets (5 oz.)
- Linguine (10 oz.)
- Tomato sauce (1 small can or 1/3 cup)
- Optional: Red pepper
- Salt and black pepper (to your liking)
- Freshly chopped parsley (.25 cup)

Preparation Guidelines:
1. Devein the shrimp and discard the shells.
2. Prepare the linguine in boiling - salted water in a large pot until al dente.
3. Warm the oil in a large skillet. Mince and add the garlic to sauté until brown. (Add red pepper, if desired.)
4. Mix in the white wine and clams. Put a lid on the pan and cook for about five minutes using the med-high temperature setting. Discard the top from the pan and simmer for another minute.
5. Pour in the tomato sauce with a sprinkle of pepper and salt.
6. Fold in the rest of the seafood, stir it, and continue cooking until the mussels and clams open.
7. Shake the parsley in with linguine.
8. Notes: Select any variety of seafood that's available in your location.
☐

Penne Rustica

Servings: 8| **Difficulty**: Medium | **Time**: 35-40 minutes

Ingredients Needed:

The Gratinata Sauce:
- Butter (3 tbsp.)
- Garlic (2 tbsp.)
- Shallot (1)
- Marsala wine (3 tbsp.)
- Heavy cream (2 cups)
- Parmesan cheese (1 cup - grated)
- Milk (not skim (.5 cup)
- Chicken broth (.5 cup)
- Cornstarch (1 tbsp.)
- Freshly minced rosemary (2 tsp.)
- Salt (.5 tsp.)
- Dijon mustard (1 tbsp.)
- Freshly minced thyme (.5 tsp.)
- Ground cayenne pepper (.5 tsp.)

The Penne Layer:
- Mini penne or ziti pasta (1 lb.)
- Shrimp (12 medium)
- Butter (2 tbsp.) can sub. 1 tbsp. each-butter+olive oil
- Grilled or smoked chicken breast - in strips (1 lb.)
- Thick-sliced smoked prosciutto, chopped (2 oz.)
- Parmesan cheese (3 tbsp. - grated)
- Paprika (1.5 tsp.)
- Pimento (12 slices)
- *Also Needed*: 9 x 11 or similar size

Preparation Guidelines:
1. Prepare the gratinata sauce by melting three tablespoons of butter in a saucepan using the low-temperature setting.
2. Mince and add the garlic and shallot. Sauté them for one to two minutes using the low-temperature setting. Stir in the marsala wine and simmer for five minutes.
3. Whisk in the rest of the fixings and let it simmer until the sauce thickens.*
4. Transfer the pan to the countertop to slightly cool. Once it is room temperature, pop it into the fridge until ready to make the dish.
5. Prepare the pasta layer. Cook the pasta until it's al dente, drain it into a colander, and spritz it with oil. Set it to the side for now.
6. Spray the baking dish with cooking oil spray.
7. Dust the shrimp with the cajun. Toss it into a sauté pan with butter/oil and cook until it's no longer pink (don't overcook). Chop the shrimp into bite-size pieces, and set aside.
8. Combine three tablespoons of parmesan with 1.5 teaspoons of paprika (set aside).
9. Warm the oven at 500° Fahrenheit.
10. Do the prep. Toss the pasta into a container. Chop and add the chicken, shrimp, and prosciutto. Pour in the gratinata sauce and stir.
11. Pour the pasta into a baking dish, tucking the pimento strips into the top of the dish.
12. Pour gratinata sauce over the entire mixture. Sprinkle the parmesan/paprika mixture on top.
13. Bake until the top begins to brown and the fixings begin to bubble at the edges (10 min.).
14. *The sauce takes roughly 10 minutes to thicken.

Chapter 8: NYC Restaurant Favorites

Brunch Options
Carmines Italian Salad

Servings: 2-4 | **Difficulty**: Easy | **Time**: 30-35 minutes

Ingredients Needed:
- Iceberg lettuce (half of 1 medium)
- Radicchio - leaf chicory (1 medium head)
- Watercress (2 bunches or Arugula (2-3 bunches)
- Genoa salami (.5 cup)
- Mortadella (.5 cup)
- Provolone (.5 cup)
- Red onion (half of 1 medium)
- Small cucumber (half of 1 small)
- Pepperoncini peppers (5)
- Pitted green olives (5 large)
- Kalamata/Gaeta pitted black olives (5)
- Radishes (3)
- Ripe tomato (1 large)
- Vinaigrette (.25 to .5 cup)
- Dried oregano (1 pinch)
- Black pepper & salt (to your liking)

Preparation Guidelines:
1. Do most of the prep before you begin. Coarsely chop the salami and mortadella. Dice the provolone. Peel and thinly slice the red onion. Peel and chop the cucumber into small chunks. Trim and thinly slice the radishes. Core and slice the tomato into eight wedges.
2. Use a sharp knife to slice the iceberg lettuce into three sections, then cut each one of them into quarters. Toss it into a container of ice-cold water.
3. Core and slice the radicchio in half. Section it into three sections and toss it into the container.
4. Discard the stems from the arugula/watercress and add them to the bowl.
5. Spin/dry the greens and toss to break them apart. Store them in the fridge to crisp.
6. Toss all of the salad fixings and pour about ¼ cup of the vinaigrette over the salad.
7. Garnish the delicious salad with oregano, salt, pepper, and dressing as desired. Serve with tomato wedges.

Sicilian Pepperoni Pizza at Prince Street Pizza

Servings: 8 by 13-inch pizza | **Difficulty**: Medium | **Time**: varies

Ingredients Needed:
- 72-hour dough (1 batch - below)
- Tomato sauce - Spicy Sicilian variation of choice (1 cup)
- Thinly sliced pepperoni (3 oz.)
- Fresh mozzarella (4 oz.)
- Shredded fontina (4 oz.)
- Olive oil (.25 cup)
- Fine sea salt and pepper (as desired)

Preparation Guidelines:
1. Warm the oven at 500° Fahrenheit for one hour.
2. Arrange the pizza dough ball on a lightly oiled sheet tray. Lightly drizzle it with oil and cover with plastic wrap. Set it aside for two to five hours until it puffs up slightly.
3. Discard the plastic wrap, and gently press the dough over the pizza tray. Spritz a little more oil over the top of dough and dust it using sea salt and pepper.
4. Scatter the tomato sauce, cheese, and pepperoni over the crust - leaving about one inch around the perimeter for the crust.
5. Set a timer and bake for ten minutes. At that time, open the oven and rotate the sheet tray 180 degrees. Bake for another five minutes or until the cheese until it's browned to your liking.
6. Remove the tray from the oven and cool it on top of a wire rack for five minutes.
7. Cut into the desired shapes and serve.
☐

Spicy Honey Soppressata Pizza "The Bee Sting Pizza" at Roberta's Pizzeria

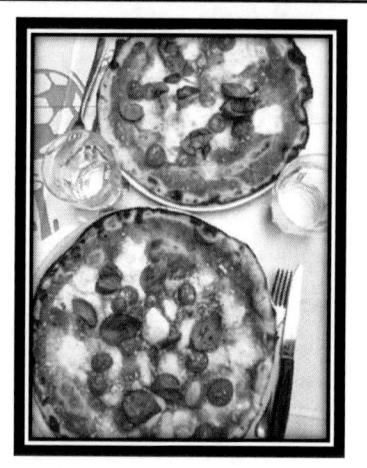

Servings: 2 | **Difficulty**: Easy | **Time**: 20 minutes

Ingredients Needed:
- Pizza dough - room temperature (16 oz.)
- Pizza sauce (.33 to .5 cup)
- Freshly torn mozzarella (6 oz.)
- Hot soppressata (8 slices)
- Basil leaves (6-8)
- For the Drizzle: Honey

Preparation Guidelines:
1. Arrange a pizza stone on the lowest rack in the oven. Set the oven at 500° Fahrenheit.
2. Lightly dust flour on a pizza peel. Working quickly, dust pizza dough in flour and stretch gently into a thin circle shape. Depending on the size of your pizza, spread one-third to one-half cup pizza sauce in a thin, even layer across the dough.
3. Tear and place the mozzarella cheese onto the pizza crust.
4. With a quick jerk motion, the pizza should quickly release from the peel onto the pizza stone in the oven.
5. Bake the pizza in the oven for about ten minutes.
6. Transfer the pan to the countertop and prepare it with a drizzle of honey, and freshly chopped basil leaves.
7. Slice and serve.

Dinner Options

<u>*Carmine's Baked Clams*</u>

Servings: 2-3| **Difficulty**: Easy | **Time**: 35-40 minutes

Ingredients Needed:
- Little Neck clams (1 dozen)
- Bottled clam juice (1 cup)
- Breadcrumbs (.75 cup)
- Garlic (1 tbsp.)
- Olive oil (1 tbsp.)
- Lemons (2 halved)
- Grated Romano cheese

Preparation Guidelines:
1. Warm the oven at 400
2. Rinse and scrub the clams. Open them up to loosen the muscle underneath the meat of the clam. Leave the clam and juices in the bottom half of the shell.
3. Place the clams in an oven-proof tray or another shallow baking pan.
4. Spoon about four teaspoons of the clam juice over each of the clams.
5. Smash one teaspoon of the breadcrumbs over each one and layer with the minced garlic. Dust with the grated cheese and a spritz of oil.
6. Bake the clams for 15 minutes until it's crispy. Lastly, broil the clams another two to three minutes.
7. Spoon the extra sauce over the clams and serve with a lemon half.

Carmine's Chicken Parmigiana

Servings: 2-3 | **Difficulty**: Easy |
Time: Cooking time is 40 min./up to 3.5 hours - varies

Ingredients Needed:
- Flour (1 cup)
- Eggs (2 large)
- Breadcrumbs (3 cups)
- Chicken breasts - ¼-inch thickness (two 5-oz. each)
- Freshly cracked black pepper & salt
- Vegetable oil (.5 cup)
- Marinara sauce (2 cups)
- Thick slices mozzarella cheese (7 oz./5-6 slices ¼-inch)
- Grated Romano cheese (2 tbsp.)

Preparation Guidelines:
1. Warm the oven at 450° Fahrenheit or optionally use the broiler (your choice).
2. Place the chicken in between layers of waxed paper. Use a mallet to flatten them until they're ¼-inch thick.
3. Prepare three containers; one with flour in a platter, whisked eggs in a bowl, and breadcrumbs on a baking tray.
4. First, sprinkle the cutlets with pepper and salt. Dip them in the flour, egg mixture, and breadcrumbs. Shake off the excess in each step.
5. Pop them in the fridge on a plate to chill for two to three hours.
6. Prepare a large sauté pan to warm the oil using the medium-temperature setting.
7. Fry the chicken for about three minutes per side and place it on a layer of paper towels.
8. Warm a saucepan (med-high temperature setting) to prepare the sauce for four to five minutes.
9. Arrange them in a casserole dish with the mozzarella on top and sprinkle of grated cheese.

10. Bake them for three to four minutes to melt the cheese (broiler time two to three minutes).
11. Serve with a spoon of sauce on a platter, add the cutlets and sauce over the top.

Spicy Vodka Rigatoni at Mario Carbone's

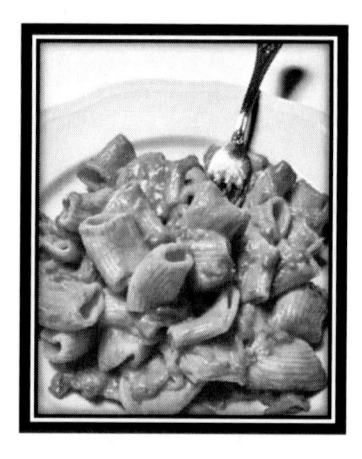

Servings: 8 | **Difficulty**: Medium | **Time**: 30 minutes

Ingredients Needed:
- Brown onions (3)
- Water (.5 cup)
- Unsalted butter (4 tbsp.)
- Salt

The Rigatoni:
- Whole tomatoes - hand crushed - ex. San Marzano (28 oz. can)
- Salt (1 tbsp./as desired)
- Sugar (2 tbsp.)
- Olive oil (3 tbsp.)
- Calabrian chili paste (1-2 tbsp.)
- Vodka** (3 tbsp.)
- •Heavy cream/as desired (1-2 cups)
- Unsalted butter (3 tbsp.)
- Rigatoni or pipette (1 lb.)

Preparation Guidelines:
1. Drain the juices from the tomatoes if you prefer a thicker sauce - before crushing them.
2. Make the onion soubise. Warm a saucepan using the low-temperature setting to melt the butter. Slice and add the onions, water, and salt. Simmer for about 15 minutes, occasionally stirring until the onions are softened and translucent.
3. Meanwhile, prepare a large skillet and combine the tomatoes, salt, sugar, olive oil, Calabrian chili paste, vodka, butter, and cream. Wait for it to boil and adjust the temperature setting to med-low. Simmer the mixture for 15-20 minutes.
4. Meanwhile, boil the pasta in a pot of salted water per the package directions (8-10 min. approx.), reserving one cup of pasta water. Drain the pasta and set it aside.
5. Add the onion soubise to the sauce and stir until thoroughly mixed. Adjust the seasoning to taste.
6. Combine the cooked pasta and two tablespoons of the pasta water, tossing to coat, and, if needed, adding more pasta water (2 tbsp. at a time) to achieve the desired sauce consistency.
7. Serve in warm bowls and when it's as you like it.
8. Note: **You can omit the vodka if desired.

Chapter 9: The Old Spaghetti Factory

Brunch Options
<u>Chicken Tetrazzini</u>

Servings: 10-12 | **Difficulty**: Easy | **Time**: 1.5 hours

Ingredients Needed:
- Uncooked spaghetti (16 oz. pkg.)
- Butter (2 tbsp.)
- Green pepper (1 medium)
- Onion (1 medium)
- Cubed chicken (2 cups - cooked)
- Mushrooms (2 cans - 4 oz. each)
- Diced pimiento (2 oz. jar)
- Condensed cream of mushrooms soup - undiluted (10.75 oz. can)
- Milk (2 cups)
- Garlic powder (.5 tsp.)
- Salt (.5 tsp.)
- Shredded cheddar cheese (4-6 oz./1.5 cups)

Preparation Guidelines:
1. Cook the spaghetti per the directions provided on the package.
2. Melt the butter in a dutch oven.
3. Dice and sauté the onions and peppers until they're tender.
4. Drain the mushrooms and pimento in a colander. Dice the chicken into chunks. Fold in the rest of the fixings (mushrooms, chicken, soup, pimiento, garlic powder, salt, and milk).
5. Drain the spaghetti and combine it with the sauce.
6. Cover and bake for 50 minutes to an hour until bubbly.
7. Remove the cover, sprinkle with cheese, and bake until the cheese is nicely browned (10 min.).

Spaghetti With Burnt Butter

Servings: 4 | **Difficulty**: Easy | **Time**: 60 minutes

Ingredients Needed:
- Butter (1 cup)
- Mizithra cheese (.5 cup - shredded)
- Parmesan cheese (.5 cup - shredded)
- Spaghetti/pasta of choice

Preparation Guidelines:
1. Dice the butter into chunks and place them in a two-quart saucepan to melt using the medium-temperature setting (5 min.).
2. Cook the butter until it's amber in color (1-2 min.). Remove the pan from the burner and wait a few minutes for the sediment to settle to the bottom of the pan.
3. Pour the brown butter through a strainer into a small bowl, leaving it undisturbed. Use the top part of the butter (clarified) and leave the sediments collected in the bottom of the pan.
4. Store the butter in the refrigerator. Use a microwave to heat it as needed.
5. Boil the pasta and drain it into a colander. Add it to four dishes and add the cheese and hot brown butter.

Dinner Option
Beer Chili

Servings: 6-8 | **Difficulty**: Super Easy | **Time**: 40 minutes

Ingredients Needed:
- Ground beef (1 lb.)
- Onion (1 small)
- Green pepper (1)
- Undrained kidney beans (1 can)
- Chili beans in sauce (1 can)
- Tomato sauce (8 oz. can)
- Diced tomatoes (14.5 oz. can)
- Apple cider vinegar (1 tbsp.)
- Chili powder (2 tbsp.)
- Chipotle chili powder (.5 to 1 tsp.)
- Garlic powder (.5 tsp.)
- Salt (.5 tsp.)
- Sugar 1 tsp.)
- Beer (8-10 oz./as desired)

Preparation Guidelines:
1. Prep the veggies by chopping the onions and pepper.
2. Brown the beef, green pepper, and onion in a skillet until done and the veggies are softened. Drain the juices and add the rest of the fixings to the pan.
3. Once boiling, adjust the temperature setting to simmer - occasionally stirring (20 min.).
4. Portion the chili into serving dishes with a portion of sour cream, chopped onions, chives, and shredded cheese. The Warehouse also used this delicious chili over its spaghetti!
☐

Sauce Favorite
Creamy Pesto Salad Dressing

Servings: 2.5 cups | **Difficulty**: Super-Easy | **Time**: 5 minutes

Ingredients Needed:
- Mayonnaise (1 cup)
- Buttermilk - low-fat (1.25 cups)
- Garlic powder (.5 tsp.)
- Freshly cracked black pepper & salt (1/8 tsp. each)
- Dried basil (1.5 tbsp.)
- Finely grated parmesan cheese (.25 cup)

Preparation Guidelines:
1. Toss all of the fixings into a mixing container.
2. Whisk until it's creamy. Pour it into a closed container.
3. Store it in the fridge for about one hour for the flavors to meld.
4. Use the delicious dressing as a dip or with a salad.

Chapter 10: Zio's Italian Kitchen

Brunch Options
Chicken Pepperoni

Servings: 4-6 | **Difficulty**: Easy | **Time**: 20 minutes

Ingredients Needed:
- Chicken breasts (1.5 lb. - boneless & skinless)
- Sliced pepperoni (4-6 oz.)
- Marinara - Bertolli/your preference (1 jar)
- Penne pasta (1 lb.)
- Sweet onion (1 large)
- Green & yellow bell pepper (1 large of each)
- Fresh mushrooms (8 oz.)
- Garlic (3 tbsp.)
- Black olives (1 small can - drained)
- Red pepper flakes (1 tsp.)
- Olive oil
- Shredded mozzarella cheese (8 oz.)
- _Optional_: Grated Romano or Parmesan cheese

Preparation Guidelines:
1. Pour four quarts of water and salt on to boil in a six-quart pot. Once the water is boiling, add in the pasta.
2. Chop or julienne the onions and peppers. Thick slice the mushrooms.
3. Prepare a hot skillet, add two teaspoons of olive oil, and sauté the mushrooms, onions, peppers, and pepperoni. Dice and add the olives, garlic, and chicken, stirring frequently.
4. Once the chicken is white, remove the pan from the burner.

5. Drain pasta when done.
6. Combine the pasta, meat mixture, grated mozzarella, and marinara; toss lightly. Top with grated parmesan/Romano cheese as desired and serve promptly.
☐

Tomato Florentine Soup

Servings: 6 | **Difficulty**: Medium | **Time**: 1 hour 15-20 minutes

Ingredients Needed:
- Butter - divided (3 tbsp. + 2 tbsp.)
- Flour (3 tbsp.)
- Onion (.75 cup)
- Fresh garlic (2 tbsp.)
- Chicken bouillon (3 cubes)
- Boiling water (1 cup)
- Crushed tomatoes (28 oz. can)
- Ketchup (1 tbsp.)
- Vegetable juice (.75 cup)
- Dried basil (.5 tbsp.)
- Dried dill (2 tbsp.)
- Hot pepper sauce (.25 tsp.)
- Dry white wine (2 tbsp.)
- Sugar (.5 tsp.)
- Black pepper (.25 tbsp.)
- Heavy cream (2 cups)
- Fresh spinach - julienne cut (.5 cup)

Preparation Guidelines:
1. Prepare a roux by warming three tablespoons butter in a heavy saucepan using the medium-temperature setting until it's foaming. Whisk in the flour and simmer until it's straw-colored (3 min.), and set aside to cool.
2. Dice and sauté the onions in two tablespoons butter over medium heat until they're golden brown. Mince and add the garlic and continue to sauté them for one to two minutes. Scoop the veggies into a food processor and puree.
3. Dissolve the chicken bouillon cubes in hot water.
4. Prepare a heavy pot to warm the vegetable juice, tomatoes, ketchup, and chicken base using the med-low heat setting. Stir in the pureed onion mixture, basil, dill, sugar, black pepper, hot pepper sauce, and wine. Simmer for 15 minutes. Whisk in the roux and simmer using the med-low temperature setting for another half an hour.
5. Remove the pan from the burner and whisk in the cream. Stir and fold in the spinach. Serve promptly for the best results.
☐

Dinner Option
Chicken Pomodoro

Servings: 1 | **Difficulty**: Easy | **Time**: 30 minutes

Ingredients Needed:
- Olive oil (1 oz.)
- Garlic (1 tsp.)
- Red pepper flakes (1 pinch)
- Italian marinated chicken, cooked (4 oz.)
- White wine (1 oz.)
- Fresh basil (1 tbsp.)
- Diced Roma tomatoes (2 oz.)
- Linguine pasta - cooked (9 oz.)
- Grated parmesan cheese (.25 cup)

Preparation Guidelines:
1. Prepare a skillet with oil. Mince and sauté the garlic and add with the pepper flakes, chicken, and basil until hot.
2. Stir in the tomatoes and deglaze the pan with the white wine.
3. Fold in the linguine and cheese, tossing thoroughly to serve.

Sides

Artichoke Spinach Dip

Servings: 6 | **Difficulty**: Easy | **Time**: 35-40 minutes

Ingredients Needed:
- Freshly spinach (.75 cup)
- Unchilled cream cheese (3 oz.)
- Butter (2 tbsp.)
- Olive oil (1 tbsp.)
- Yellow onion (.25 cup)
- Flour (2 tbsp.)
- Salt (.25 tsp.)
- Half & Half (1 cup)
- Parmesan/Asiago cheese (.33 cup)
- Monterey jack cheese (1 cup - shredded)
- Mozzarella cheese (.5 cup - shredded)
- Artichokes - marinated (8 oz. jar)
- Reserved artichoke juice (.25 cup)
- Fresh lemon juice (2 tsp.)
- Real bacon bits (1.5 tbsp.)
- *To Garnish*: Roma tomato (1 diced)

Preparation Guidelines:
1. Shred all of the cheese (mozzarella, Monterey, & parmesan)and set them aside, or purchase them pre-shredded.
2. Prepare a saucepan and melt the butter using the med-low temperature setting.
3. Whisk in the salt and flour until it turns into a thick paste; don't brown. Slowly, add in the Half & Half, stirring until it thickens slightly.
4. Drain the juices from the artichokes, reserving the liquid. Stir in the Monterey Jack, parmesan, cream cheese, mozzarella (¼ cup), chopped onions, and artichokes.
5. Stir cheese mixture until thoroughly heated and mix in the reserved (¼ cup) artichoke juice and lemon juice.
6. Fold in the freshly chopped spinach and bits of bacon. Simmer until it is thoroughly blended and the mixture starts to lightly bubble.
7. Transfer it into an oiled shallow casserole dish. Sprinkle the remainder of mozzarella cheese on top.
8. Warm the oven to 350° Fahrenheit.
9. Bake it for 15-20 minutes. Once it's ready, garnish it using a portion of diced tomato and serve with a tasty crusty garlic bread or Focaccia.
☐

Bread Dipping Oil

Servings: Varies | **Difficulty**: Easy | **Time**: 5 minutes

Ingredients Needed:
Salt (1 tsp.)
- Virgin olive oil (.25 cup)

Spices: 1 tbsp. each:
- Dried basil
- Crushed red pepper flakes
- Garlic powder
- Dried rosemary
- Dried parsley
- Ground black pepper
- Dried oregano
- Dried minced garlic

Preparation Guidelines:
1. Grind all of the fixings using a coffee/spice grinder (omit the oil).
2. Measure and toss two teaspoons of the spices onto a small serving plate.
3. Drizzle/pour a thin layer of olive oil over the mixture and serve with your favorite crispy bread.

Italian Nachos

Servings: 4-6 | **Difficulty**: Easy | **Time**: 40-45 minutes

Ingredients Needed:
- Wonton wrappers (¼ of a package)
- Pepperoni (½ of a package)
- Italian sweet sausage links (2)
- Sugar (.25 cup)
- Balsamic vinegar (1 cup)
- Grated parmesan cheese (as desired)
- Whipping cream (2 cups)
- Flour (1 tbsp.)
- Cornstarch (1 tbsp.)
- Butter (2 tbsp.)
- Green onions (3 chopped)
- Kalamata olives (10 - sliced in half)
- Banana peppers (5 sliced)
- Shredded Monterey or Colby cheese (1 cup)

Preparation Guidelines:
1. Prepare a large pan to fry the wonton wrappers. Slice the wrappers diagonally into triangles. Fry them for 30 seconds in hot oil. Drain them onto paper towels once cooked. Slice the pepperoni into quarters or halves and set aside.
2. Slice the sausage links into thin rounds and slice into halves. Slowly cook them in a skillet until done.
3. Pour the cream into the pan and add shredded parmesan. Cook until all of the cheese is melted (20 min.).
4. Make the alfredo sauce with cornstarch if needed. Set this aside.
5. Make the balsamic syrup by tossing the butter into a pan, adding flour to make a rue. Pour in the vinegar and sugar; simmer until thickened.
6. Arrange the cooked wontons on a baking tray and sprinkle with the meats, olives, peppers, drizzle a cup of Alfredo Sauce.
7. Garnish with a drizzle of the balsamic syrup (4 tbsp.) and a sprinkle of the Monterey cheese. Broil them until the cheese is melted (1 min.). Top with chopped green onions and serve.

Zio's Spice Mix

Servings: 4 | Difficulty: Easy | Time: 10 minutes

Ingredients Needed:
- Red pepper flakes (1 tsp.)
- Garlic powder (1 tbsp.)
- Crushed dried rosemary (1 tbsp.)
- Dried oregano (1 tbsp.)
- Parsley (1 tsp.)
- Salt & ground pepper (.5 tsp.each)
- Dried basil (2 tsp.)
- *Optional*: Grated parmesan

Preparation Guidelines:
1. Measure and toss each of the spices into a closed container.
2. Store them for up to six weeks.
3. Add a bit of parmesan if desired.

Chapter 11: Variety Restaurants – Copycat Recipes

You will be pleasantly surprised at the list of suggestions in this segment. Enjoy each one!

Brunch Options

Godfather's Antipasto Salad/Party Tray

Servings: 1 | **Difficulty**: Easy | **Time**: 15-20 minutes

Ingredients Needed:
- *The Dressing*:
  - ✓ Olive oil (.75 cup)
  - ✓ Honey (1 tbsp.)
  - ✓ Red wine vinegar (.25 cup)
  - ✓ Dijon mustard (2 tbsp.)
  - ✓ Black pepper (.25 tsp.)
  - ✓ Salt (1 tsp.)

- *The Salad*:
  - ✓ Each Serving: Romaine & Iceberg - mixed (2 cups)

- *As Desired*:
  - ✓ Sliced salami
  - ✓ Marinated artichoke hearts
  - ✓ Thinly sliced white onion
  - ✓ Sliced mozzarella cheese
  - ✓ Halved cherry tomatoes
  - ✓ Ripe black olives
  - ✓ Optional: Garbanzo beans

Preparation Guidelines:
1. Prepare the salad according to how many people will be dining.
2. Toss the fixings for the dressing into a sealable container and shake until thoroughly mixed.
3. Arrange the cheese and salami on the plate - alternating for a fancy appearance.
4. Fill the center with the lettuce combo, quartered artichoke hearts, tomatoes, sliced onion, garbanzo beans, and olives.
5. Garnish with the jar of dressing or serve it on the side.

Godfather's Deep Dish Pizza

Servings: 6 | **Difficulty**: Experienced | **Time**: 2 hours

Ingredients Needed:
- Diced tomatoes (28 oz. can)
- Italian sausage (1 lb.)
- Rapid-rise active yeast (0.25 oz. pkg.)
- Granulated sugar (1 tsp.)
- Warm water (1 cup)
- Yellow cornmeal (.5 cup)
- Flour (2.5 cups)
- Olive oil (.25 cup)
- Shredded mozzarella cheese (1 lb.)
- Dried oregano (1 tsp.)
- Dried sweet basil (1 tsp.)
- Grated parmesan cheese (.5 cup)

Preparation Guidelines:
1. Drain the tomatoes and set aside. Cook the sausage and set it aside.
2. Whisk the warm water (105-115° Fahrenheit), yeast, and sugar in a mixing container.
3. Fold in two cups of the flour, salt, cornmeal, and olive oil.
4. Use the paddle and mix on speed '2' for two minutes.
5. Put on the dough hook and add the remaining flour. Knead on speed '2' until the dough clings to the hook.
6. Knead on speed '2' for another five minutes. Arrange the dough in a greased mixing container and cover. Place the bowl in a warm space and leave it to rise for one hour.
7. Warm the oven at 500° Fahrenheit.
8. Press the dough into a deep-dish pizza pan using oiled hands to keep it from sticking to you. Cover the dough with the mozzarella. Crumble and add the sausage, diced tomatoes, oregano, basil, and parmesan cheese.
9. Bake it for 15 minutes.
10. Adjust the temperature setting to 350° Fahrenheit and bake until the crust is brown (20 min.).

Uno's Chicago Grill Shrimp Scampi Pasta

Servings: 4 | **Difficulty**: Easy | **Time**: 30 minutes

Ingredients Needed:
- Garlic (1 tbsp.)
- Olive oil (1 oz.)
- Cooked shrimp - tail off (4 oz.)
- Seasoned plum tomatoes (.25 cup - see below)
- Fresh basil (1 tsp.)
- White wine (1 oz.)
- Scampi butter sauce (5 oz.)
- Cooked pasta (12 oz.)

Preparation Guidelines:
1. Make the seasoned tomatoes. Chop the tomatoes, basil, oregano, and garlic butter.
2. Make the butter sauce in a sauté pan. Combine the seafood stock, butter, lemon, basil, garlic, and onion. Use the medium-temperature setting to warm the oil, stirring in the garlic mix, sautéing it briefly - but do not brown.
3. Mix in the tomatoes, shrimp, and basil. Toss, sauté, and mix in the scampi sauce and let it heat two to three minutes.
4. Fold in the well-drained pasta and serve.

Dinner Options
Taco Pizza by Pizza Inn

Servings: 2 | **Difficulty**: Super-Easy | **Time**: 30-35 minutes

Ingredients Needed:
- Pizza crust (1)
- Ground beef (.5 lb.)
- Refried beans (1 small can)
- Taco seasoning (half of 1 pkg.)
- Crispy lettuce
- Freshly diced tomatoes
- Shredded cheddar cheese

Preparation Guidelines:
1. Set the oven at 350° Fahrenheit with a pizza stone inside.
2. Have the pizza peel ready. You can use a prepared crust or choose to make one from scratch.
3. Brown and crumble the beef in a skillet. Drain the fat/juices, add water, and the taco seasoning.
4. After the crust is partially baked (10 min.), place it on top of the stove and add the refried beans over the pie shell (leaving a ½-inch rim).
5. Scatter the crumbled beef over the top. Place the prepared pizza onto a pizza stone. Bake it until ingredients on top are thoroughly heated (10-15 min.). Take the pizza pan out of the oven and top generously with lettuce, tomatoes, and cheddar cheese. Serve with a smile!

Sides

Papa John's Garlic Knots

Servings: 16 | **Difficulty**: Super-Easy | **Time**: 25 minutes

Ingredients Needed:
- Melted - unsalted butter (.25 cup)
- Garlic powder (.75 tsp.)
- Dried parsley flakes (.5 tsp.)
- Freshly grated Parmesan (2 tbsp.)
- Dried oregano (.5 tsp.)
- Salt (.25 tsp.)
- Refrigerated buttermilk biscuits (16 oz. tube)

Preparation Guidelines:
1. Set the oven at 400° Fahrenheit.
2. Spritz a baking tray with a layer of cooking oil spray.
3. Whisk the parmesan, butter, garlic powder, parsley, salt, and oregano in a small mixing container. Set it to the side for now.
4. Slice each of the eight biscuits to make 16 knots. Roll each chunk into a five-inch rope (½-inch thick). Tie it in a knot and tuck in the ends.
5. Brush each of the prepared garlic knots with about half of the butter. Arrange them on the baking tray.
6. Bake them until they are nicely browned (8-10 min.). Serve promptly - brushed with the rest of the butter mixture.

The Spaghetti Warehouse Meat Sauce

Servings: 6-8 | Difficulty: Super-Easy | Time: 2.5 hours

Ingredients Needed:
- Onions (2)
- Oil (1 tbsp.)
- Ground beef (2 lb.)
- Italian seasoning (1 tbsp.)
- Garlic powder (1 tbsp.)
- Salt (1 tsp.)
- Pepper (.5 tsp.)
- Stewed tomatoes (28 oz. can)
- Tomato paste (2 cans @ 5.5 oz. each)
- Garlic cloves (4)
- *Optional*: White wine/Vermouth (.25 cup)

Preparation Guidelines:
1. Dice and sauté the onions. Toss in the beef and simmer until it's browned.
2. Add the seasonings, cloves, paste, and tomatoes.
3. Stir in the alcohol (if using) and cover.
4. Simmer with a lid on the pot using the low-temperature setting for at least two hours.
5. Serve when it's ready as desired.
☐

Desserts

Ci Ci's Cherry Dessert Pizza

Servings: 8 | **Difficulty**: Super-Easy | **Time**: 40-45 minutes

Ingredients Needed:
- *The Pizza*:
  ✓ Cherry pie filling (20 oz. can)
  ✓ Pizza mix (1 pkg.)
  ✓ Crumb topping (.25 cup)

- *The Topping*:
  ✓ Brown sugar (1 tbsp.)
  ✓ Flour (.5 cup)
  ✓ Sugar (3 tbsp.)
  ✓ Softened butter (.25 cup)
  ✓ Salt (1/8 tsp.)

Preparation Guidelines:
1. Warm the oven to reach 450° Fahrenheit. Lightly spritz a pizza pan with cooking oil spray.
2. Prepare the pizza dough per the package instructions and spread it onto the prepared pan. Prick it with a fork eight to ten times. Place the pan in the hot oven to bake for five minutes.
3. Transfer the cooked crust from the oven and add the pie filling over the hot crust. Sprinkle it with ¼ of a cup of crumb topping and bake for another 20 to 25 minutes. Remove the pizza when the dough is golden brown.
4. Prepare the topping. Whisk the dry fixings (flour, sugar, brown sugar, and salt). Combine all of the components until the topping resembles cornmeal.

Ci Ci's Chocolate Dessert Pizza

Servings: 8 | **Difficulty**: Easy | **Time**: 35 minutes

Ingredients Needed:
- *The Pizza*:
  - Pizza dough mix (1 pkg.)
  - Chocolate pudding mix - cooked & cooled (3.4 oz. box)

- *The Mix*:
  - Sugar (3 tbsp.)
  - Flour (.5 cup)
  - Salt (1/8 tsp.)
  - Brown sugar (1 tbsp.)
  - Softened butter (.25 cup)

Note: The pudding mix should be the cooked type - not instant.

Preparation Guidelines:
1. Warm the oven at 450° Fahrenheit.
2. Prepare the pizza dough per the package instructions.
3. Stretch and shape the dough on a greased pizza pan. Pierce the dough with a fork eight to ten times. Bake for about five minutes.
4. Remove the pan from the oven and spread ¾ of a cup of chocolate pudding over the dough and sprinkle with ¼ of a cup of the crumb topping. Pop it back in the oven and bake until it's crispy (18-20 min.).
5. Mix the flour, sugar, salt, and brown sugar. Blend in the butter until it resembles cornmeal.

Godfather's Pizza: Cinnamon Streusel Dessert Pizza

Servings: 3-4 or 8 slices | **Difficulty**: Easy | **Time**: 25 minutes

Ingredients Needed:
- Pizza dough (homemade or store-bought)
- Melted butter (1 tbsp.)
- Cinnamon

- *The Streusel*:
✓ A-P flour (1/2 cup + 1/3 cup)
✓ White sugar (1/3 cup)
✓ Olive oil (2 tbsp.)
✓ Vegetable shortening (2 tbsp.)
✓ Brown sugar (.25 cup)

- *The Icing*:
✓ Powdered sugar (1 cup)
✓ Milk (1 tbsp.)
✓ Vanilla (.5 tsp.)
✓ Also Needed: 12-inch pizza pan

Preparation Guidelines:
1. Whisk the streusel ingredients and set side aside. Lightly spritz the pizza pan using a cooking oil spray.
2. Pat the dough into the pan. "Poke" the dough with a fork to reduce air bubbles while baking. Melt one tablespoon of butter and brush the dough. Sprinkle cinnamon all around the buttered crust. Top the pizza crust with the streusel mix.
3. Bake at 460° Fahrenheit for eight to nine minutes.
4. Combine the icing fixings until it has a drizzle consistency.
5. Decorate the pie using the icing in a circular pinwheel pattern. Slice and serve.
☐

Beverage Favorite
The Spaghetti Warehouse Sangria

Servings: 2-4/varies | **Difficulty**: Super-Easy | **Time**: 5 minutes

Ingredients Needed:
- Brandy (1 oz.)
- Orange liquor (1 oz.)
- Orange juice (3 oz.)
- Fruit punch (9 oz.)
- Riunite Lambrusco (18 oz.)
- *Also Needed*: 64 oz. pitcher

Preparation Guidelines:
1. Fill the pitcher with ice and add each of the delicious mixers.
2. Stir well and garnish with your favorite fruit, such as cherries, oranges, lemons, or limes!

Conclusion

I hope you are geared for your new dining experience after reading each chapter of Copycat Recipes.

If you have any concerns about alcohol, put them to rest. Alcohol will start to evaporate at three times the rate of water when combined. You can speed the process by leaving the lid off the skillet/pan. (An open cover will lead to faster evaporation compared to a closed top.)

However, you will need to cook food for about three hours to erase all traces of alcohol fully. After an hour of cooking, 25% of the alcohol remains, and even after two and a half hours, there's still 5% of it.

The Italians figured it out; alcohol is versatile! Whether you use a rum, sake, or beer, alcohol is a perfect flavor enhancer, tenderizer, as a marinade, or simmered in sauces. Italians love it! The next step is to decide which dish you want to prepare first. That is the great part; you have the recipes to a ton of restaurant-style menu items to choose from for your family and friends to enjoy!

If you found this book useful and valuable for cooking your favorite recipes, I kindly ask you to leave an honest review on Amazon. I would really appreciate it! Thank you so much! :)

Manufactured by Amazon.ca
Acheson, AB